Paediatrics: What shall I do?

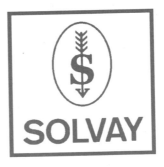

This book is provided to

....

as a service to medicine
from Solvay Healthcare

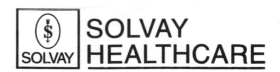

Paediatrics:

What shall I do?

Mike Liberman, MB, FRCP, DCH

Bev Daily, MB, BS

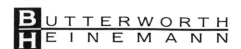

Butterworth-Heinemann Ltd
Linacre House, Jordan Hill, Oxford OX2 8DP

A member of the Reed Elsevier plc group

OXFORD LONDON BOSTON
MUNICH NEW DELHI SINGAPORE SYDNEY
TOKYO TORONTO WELLINGTON

First published 1993
Reprinted 1995

British Library Cataloguing in Publication Data
A catalogue record for this book is available from the
British Library

Library of Congress Cataloging in Publication Data
A catalogue record for this book is available from the
Library of Congress

ISBN 0 7506 1402 1

Composition by Scribe Design, Gillingham, Kent
Printed and bound in Great Britain by
Biddles Ltd, Guildford and King's Lynn

Preface

There is no situation in which the doctor is more likely to walk a tightrope than in dealing with a sick child. The busy GP sees dozens of slightly unwell children in a week. The vast majority are no more than that. Unfortunately, with few exceptions, the ones who become really sick, desperately ill, usually started off by being slightly unwell.

The comforting words, 'I am sure there's nothing to be worried about, my dear', that have sent many a mother happier to bed do not sound as good, in retrospect, when the child is sent into hospital 6 hours later, by another doctor, with meningococcal meningitis. There are few cases which reach the courts – and how many cases in the courts involve children – in which the parents have not been similarly reassured.

Added to this, there is the veterinary aspect. A 6-week-old baby does not give a particularly good history: neither, on occasion, does the mother of a 6-week-old baby. 'Burning up', 'screaming with pain', 'throwing everything up' can in turn mean a child with too many clothes on, one who is hungry, and one who is posseting.

On the other hand, both authors have seen desperately ill children about whom the parents – caring, perhaps very intelligent – have shown no alarm, or even concern, for example, the 'snuffly' child who turns out to be in severe heart failure, or the 'croaky throat' who turns out to have a bulbar palsy.

The object of this little book, therefore, is to try to sort out the kind of problems a GP, or any other doctor working with children, might encounter when the standard text book, rich in muscular dystrophies perhaps, might rather fail to address. In any case where a subject's initials are used eg. URTI, bear with us when, for those not into 'Doctor-speak', the full name is given at least once. UTI, ENT, ADH are all extremely familiar, but less so perhaps, are CMA and RAP. Also, whilst we appreciate that large numbers of children are cared for by female doctors and that the parent who brings the child to the doctor is often the father, in order to avoid confusion and the clumsy repetitive use of 'he or she' we have, invariably, called the doctor 'he' and represented the parent as the mother.

Should a febrile child have his temperature taken during the night? Can paracetamol be given more than 4 times in 24 hours? What is the best way to treat a wheezy 6-month-old baby? Should a woman stop breast feeding her baby when it has severe diarrhoea? What should she do if the baby refuses to take anything else? Do children have growing pains? Are apnoea alarms worth the hassle? What would be a precocious puberty?

These, and many other questions, are asked by a GP who has spent years pondering on such problems. They are answered by a paediatric consultant who has spent a similar length of time answering them. The book is in no way meant to cover the vast field of paediatrics, but just to offer succour to those doctors who wonder 'What shall I do?'

As has been said in other books of this series, any GP could think of hundreds more questions, nor would the same answers necessarily be given by other paediatricians. Nevertheless, they are answers, and from a background of many years of experience.

The index of this book refers to question numbers and not to page numbers so that, in extremis, a quick crib can be obtained under the light of the auriscope as the doctor leaves the patient for a moment to 'get something from the car.' It can be flicked through in those odd moments when the insurance medical hasn't turned up for his appointment, or in the lounge when the children insist on watching something educational on the television, or most relaxing of all, in the bath.

The tightrope will still exist. Perhaps this book will, at least, serve as a balancing pole.

M.L.
B.D.

Publisher's note
A number of paediatric problems such as the management of childhood epilepsy and the diagnosis of squint are covered in the companion titles to this volume, 'Neurology. What shall I do?' Thomas/Daily and 'Ophthalmology. What shall I do?' Kanski/Daily.

Contents

viii   *Contents*

Pyrexial problems

Question 1. Avoiding hyperpyrexia

A doctor is called out to see a child aged 2 years with a temperature of 103.8°F. There are no particularly abnormal physical signs and a diagnosis of 'virus infection' is made. The doctor advises paracetamol and tepid sponging. The temperature comes down and the mother is reassured. It is late evening and the child is put to bed. Should the mother disturb the child in the night to check the temperature in case he becomes hyperpyrexial in his sleep? If the temperature were checked in this way at what level would you advise the tepid sponging to be repeated?

There is no need to disturb the child. Active cooling can be carried out over 102°F.

Nearly all very feverish children have a disturbed night, waking spontaneously, or may show delirium and there is no need to rouse them intentionally. Parents need to be taught to look for the appearance of important symptoms or signs, for it is rarely the fever itself that matters but what is causing it.

The one exception is that small group of children to whom 'prophylactic' rectal diazepam is given to forestall further febrile fits. The regime sets a temperature equal to, or above 101.3°F (38.5°C) rectally at which point the rectal solution – 5 mg for a child 1–3 years, 2.5 mg if less than 1 year – should be administered and repeated every 12 hours, if temperature reaches 101.3°F or above, to a maximum of 4 times in 48 hours.

Putting the child to bed with vest and nappy, covered only with a cotton sheet – it is difficult for most children to sleep without some cover – with adequate fluid intake and a full dose of paracetamol will avoid most night-time hyperpyrexia. I consider a full dose of paracetamol to be 20 mg/kg per dose assuming a 6-hourly space between doses. In effect this can mean, for the average size 2-year-old toddler of 13 kg, a dose of paracetamol infant mixture

Table 1. Centigrade/Fahrenheit conversion table

	AXILLA	RECTAL/ORAL	98.6	99.5	100.4	101.3	102.2	103.1	
°F	97.4	98.4	99	100	101	102	103	104	105
°C	36.3	36.9	37	37.5	38	38.5	39	39.5 40	
NORMAL VALUES			37.2	37.8	38.3	38.9	39.4		40.6

(125 mg/5 ml) of 10 ml. The parents, however, may be happier to give the paracetamol more frequently, e.g. every 4 hours (see Question 4 for dosage).

Tepid sponging is not a toddler's favourite activity and, if available, a fan is better. Sponging should be used, however, if other methods fail or the fever is high (>102°F/39°C) and I would, by and large, advise active cooling above 102°F.

Thermometers, like the British, are rarely bilingual. A reference spatula in the top pocket, using the data illustrated in Table 1, may help. My experience with fever scans and electronic thermometers is unfavourable. I encourage parents to use a glass thermometer held under the child's axilla for 3 minutes. Apart from anything else, this ensures that clothes are removed and increases the chances of observing rashes and breathing difficulties, and also aids cooling. Auntie's advice to 'wrap him up warm' can rapidly microwave a pyrexial child to convulsion pitch!

Question 2. How many dry nappies constitute dehydration?

A little girl of 18 months has been unwell with a throat infection for 3 days. She has vomited on several occasions and is on antibiotics. The doctor sees the child at 2 p.m. because the mother is concerned that there has been no wet nappy since the night before. The child does not appear clinically dehydrated. Would you be concerned about this lack of urinary output? If not, how long before you did worry?

No urinary output does not necessarily mean no urinary production.

The issue to be decided is whether or not there is withholding of micturition. It is not uncommon for the toddler to hold back, having once experienced the discomfort of passing concentrated, acid urine. You might be able to palpate a full bladder. Some paracetamol and a warm bath may lead to evacuation, but I would be prepared not to interfere for up to 24 hours.

The alternative explanation is much more serious, true oliguria or anuria, and it is just possible to be deceived by significant dehydration in an alkalotic toddler brought on by considerable vomiting. A recent known weight compared to that on the bathroom scales now should reveal a significant weight loss, say, of 10% body weight.

If in doubt, encourage fluids, 15 ml every 15 minutes for 2 hours. If the child refuses or vomits admit to hospital, when an ultrasound can quickly assess an empty/full bladder.

Question 3. To bed or not to bed?

A child of 5 years is hot and unwell but does not want to go to bed, preferring to lie by the fire and watch 'Neighbours'. Bearing in mind that in conditions like otitis media the child would be more comfortable sitting up, should any rule apply to bed rest in children or do they instinctively know 'what's best for them'?

In the majority of cases children do know best.

Young children who are unwell need the closeness and security of a loved one in sight. They may rest on the settee or carpet with a TV or video to distract them.

An 'irritable hip', where non-weight bearing may expedite recovery, is the only condition where I attempt to encourage 'bed-rest' as described. The child's own reactions to his/her illness should dictate all else.

Question 4. Should you treat a temperature?

A woman phones the doctor to say that her child of 2 years has a feverish cold, is not particularly unwell, but has a pyrexia of 102°F. Should paracetamol be advised solely to bring down the temperature? Is there any evidence that the pyrexia accompanying the infection is a bodily defence mechanism that will hasten recovery? If a child is very hot and the effect of the paracetamol only seems to last for 4 hours, are you justified in giving more than 4 doses in 24 hours?

Pyrexia is a 'natural' defence reaction. Paracetamol is generally used well within its safety margins.

I will assume that you are too wise to let parents give you a diagnosis, but would allow them to describe observed symptoms and signs. If the cause of a fever is obvious a few questions can usually exclude sinister conditions and there is little risk in giving an antipyretic.

There is no good evidence that paracetamol masks important disease nor interferes with the body's responses to disease. There is plenty of evidence that pyrexia is a manifestation of an important defence response, e.g. interferon output and impedance of bacterial metabolism.

Large doses of paracetamol (20–25 mg/kg per dose) are needed at times but I would not advocate that dose more than 4 times in 24 hours. The standard dose (12 mg/kg per dose) could, of course, be given 4 hourly, i.e. 6 times a day if necessary.

It does mean, however, that if the parent is happier to give the drug 4 hourly, a total daily dose can be devised, e.g. a 12 kg toddler of 2 years could have 12 × 20 × 4 mg paracetamol, giving a total for the 24 hours of 960 mg or 8 × 5 ml teaspoons (120 mg) in the day. This could be split up into 4 hourly doses, say, of 10 ml, 5 ml, 5 ml, 5 ml, 10 ml and 5 ml.

Question 5. How hot before hospitalization?

It is a policy of some hospitals to admit all infants under a certain age with a pyrexia. As a general rule, is there an age/pyrexia standard that you would set for infants to be sent in by their GP?

It depends upon the circumstances.

I am reluctant to dogmatize. A paediatrically experienced GP who is fairly certain of the cause of the fever, e.g. other members of the family may have an upper respiratory tract infection, and is happy the infant is not ill, can clearly manage the situation at home.

Important to the doctor is the need to feel confident in the parents' abilities to communicate significant change. These abilities are not necessarily based on intellect as much as instinct, and tend to increase with the number of children in the family.

Against this background I teach SHOs to admit every pyrexial infant under 6 months unless the registrar or consultant has seen the infant and overidden that precaution.

Question 6. Prophylactic rectal diazepam

A doctor is called to see a child of 2 years with a pyrexia of 103.6°F. The child is irritable and a little 'twitchy'. The mother says that the child has had a febrile convulsion a year previously. She is trying to actively cool the child and has given paracetamol a short time before. Would you give rectal diazepam? How long would it be before you could safely leave the child after you had given it?

I probably would not use it in this case, but if I did I would stay for another 15 minutes unless otherwise indicated.

How do we assess the risk of recurrence of seizures in a child of 2 years? This has been a subject of much research, but with unclear results.

We have to attempt to define simple, benign febrile convulsions which seem to affect about 3% of normal children between the ages of 6 months and 5 years and then disappear. These children need to be separated (if possible) from a smaller group of children, who at the same age are more prone to 'convulsions with fever'. This latter group have a pre-convulsion history or evidence of neurodevelopmental abnormality, e.g. birth asphyxia, very low birth weight, or congenital or acquired neurological disease. This latter group can be thought of as having underlying epilepsy and are likely to go on having seizures beyond the age of 5 years. For 'simple, benign' seizures a distillation of risk factors has proved useful in predicting likely recurrence up to the age of 5 years.

These factors are:

• A history of febrile convulsions in a first degree relative (parent/sibling).
• A history of epilepsy in a first degree relative.
• Onset of first seizure before first birthday, especially in a girl.
• A 'complicated' first seizure, i.e. convulsing for longer than 15 minutes, atypical movements, e.g. focal and atypical post-ictal findings such as Todd's paralysis or repeated attacks in the first 24 hours following initial seizure.
• Attendance at a nursery (being exposed to more than average number of infections).

It has been estimated that the *subsequent* risk of a further simple seizure up to aged 5 years is:

• if all risk factors absent – approximately 12.5%
• if 1 factor only present – approximately 25%
• if 2 factors present – approximately 50%
• if 3 or more factors present – approximately 75%

All decisions on treatment plans must take into account the wishes of parents, once they are fully aware of the risks as best assessed, and with information on what available drugs have to offer. Prevention with continuous phenobarbitone or valproate has lost most advocates now, following concerns about side-effects. They may still be wanted and advised in the two higher risk categories above, especially if fevers occur so rapidly before the fit that the parents are caught 'unaware'. Currently rectal diazepam has most following, either as a rescue (to arrest a seizure) or as prophylaxis (given when fever reaches 101.3°F/38.5°C or above – see Question 1).

Even more important than information on drugs is that parents need careful instruction on how to handle a seizure, with clear understanding of the recovery position of body and head (with written pamphlet back-up). They must dial 999 if their child's seizure continues for about 5 minutes, and insert the diazepam at

that time. Contacting even the most available GP, if convulsing
continues, may delay treatment for 'status epilepticus' and the
direct route via ambulance into Accident and Emergency facilities able to deal with unpredictable events is the wiser action.

So to your specific example. Only one risk factor (that of a fit
when under 1 year of age) is detailed. I would not recommend
prophylaxis on one factor only, but I could be persuaded by fright-
ened parents. The most reassuring information here is that no
attack has appeared for 1 year. It is very uncommon to have the
second seizure after such a gap. Illnesses and fevers will have
come thick and fast in that time testing this child's lowered seizural threshold when he/she was most 'vulnerable', but 1 year later
that threshold is higher (i.e. less likely to seize)'.

It is vital to take a history and carefully scrutinize the child,
expecting to find a trivial viral illness, but excluding meningitis or
other serious disease. Assuming all seems well, I would continue
the antipyrexial activities (preferring a fan and adequate dose of
paracetamol – see Question 1), rehearse the first aid measures
described above and be certain that the mother has a 5 mg rectal
tube of diazepam available. Diazepam acts very quickly and if I
used it I would stay the 10–15 minutes necessary to reassure
myself of an explanation for the fever and that the parents were
convincingly reassured and coping. I would not normally expect
to admit a 'second' febrile fit.

Respiratory problems

Question 7. Asthma – how bad is it going to get?

It is early evening. The GP sees a child of 3 years who has a marked wheeze, but is not particularly distressed. The mother says that she is concerned as the child was very poorly the previous night, requiring nebulized salbutamol, and now, though not bad, he is worse than he was at the same time the previous evening. What features might decide the doctor to hospitalize the child there and then?

Assessment must be made of present severity, past severity and compliance.
The younger the child:

- The less predictable is the response to anti-asthma therapy.
- The more difficult the compliance.
- The more ingenious must be the method of delivery.

Asthma can appear in many forms, from the fast, shallow breather to the slow wheezer. Past history and the experience of the parent is essential: 'How often is he as bad as this?'
Medication currently being taken, both chronic and acute, must be absolutely clarified.
There are three phases in the assessment and management:

- Estimating the severity of the child's current clinical condition.
- Establishing the previous severity of the asthma and drug responses.
- Trying to ensure compliance and effective delivery.

Table 2 and Figure 1 show some of these issues in detail.
Compliance and effective delivery may be helped by observing the following:

- Inhaled medication should always be preferred.
- Few 3-year-olds effectively breathe deeply from a valved spacer.
- A multidose spacer, or a holding chamber, with masks (see Figure 2) have been shown to be the most efficient and should be tried first.
- If a nebulizer is used, a powerful compressor capable of air flows of 8–10 l/min working through a nebulized volume of 4 ml produces the best output of appropriate particles especially necessary for inhaled steroids.
- The mask of the nebulizer must be against the face with little

Table 2. Assessing the severity of a child's current clinical condition (3 years old)

Symptom/Sign	Asthma		
	Mild	Moderate	Severe
1. Speech	Can produce 'sentences'	Speaks in 'phrases'	Single words/speechless
2. Alertness	Normal restless	Agitated	Very agitated/confused
3. Breathlessness	Can walk, lie down, drink normally	Shorter or softer cry, drinking interruptedly	Has to rest; won't eat/drink
4. Accessory muscle use and suprasternal retraction	None	Mild	Severe/absent (fixed)
5. Respiratory rate (at rest) *Some react fast shallow, some slow wheezy (normal for 3 years = 20–30/min)	Normal or slightly up (>30)	40–60	>60
6. Wheeze (see 5*)	Mild, usually expiration only	Loud (intermittent)	Continuous
7. Pulse (at rest)	Normal (<110)	>110–140	>140
8. Pulsus paradoxicus (difficult to quantitate at this age)	Absent	May be detected	Often obvious

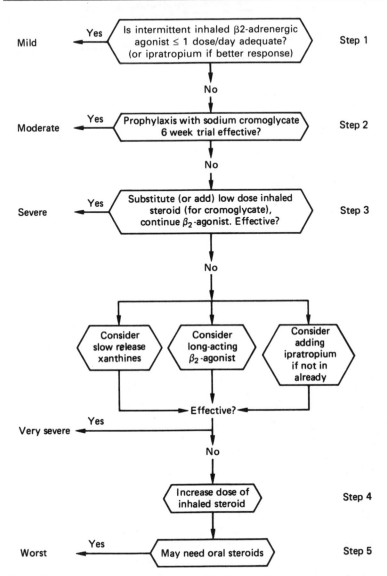

Figure 1 Assessing the previous severity of asthma and drug responses: Steps correspond to published guidelines, 1993

　dead space, or the drug delivery falls off massively for each 1 cm gap.
- Dosages must be high as nebulization only delivers a small percentage of the drug to the lungs. A metered dosage inhaler through a spacer delivers comparable amounts.

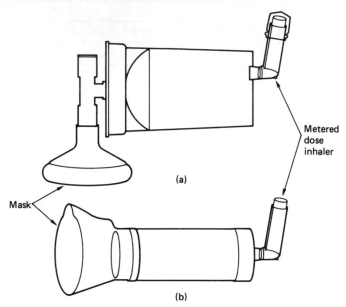

Figure 2 (a) Multidose spacer (b) Holding chamber. Each with mask

The child you have described suggests a background of moderate asthma, but the management of this exacerbation is not easy to dogmatize over. I would proceed as follows:

- Ensure the β_2-agonist and/or ipratropium is given 4 hourly (2.5 mg of salbutamol in 2.5 ml in the nebulization chamber and/or ipratropium 250 µg in 1 ml with 1 ml added *normal* saline in the nebulization chamber). If he responds well, 4 hourly nebulizers will probably be needed throughout the night or possibly a Volmax could be swallowed to spare the waking (but parents would need to check at 4-hourly intervals).
- Worsening of symptoms or signs before the next inhalation, i.e. in less than 4 hours, constitutes 'status asthmaticus' and
- Oral prednisolone (dispersible 5 mg tablets) must be available for a dosage of 2 mg/kg body weight to be given in the event of status asthmaticus.
- The child's condition must be reviewed in 4 hours – by telephone if you are confident of the parents' ability to assess and convey details accurately by telephone or preferably by the *same* doctor's full clinical reassessment.
- If steroids are used, β_2-agonists and ipratropium must be continued and the condition constantly updated (4-hourly).

- A previous history of sudden deterioration would influence me to adopt a more aggressive response here – using oral steroids and more frequent β_2-agonist and ipratropium at first contact.
- Four-hourly reviews, or sooner if the parents request, are mandatory until improvement persists and 'precautionary' admission should be sought if any doubts remain in the parents' ability to manage or the doctor's confidence to oversee. Night-time unfortunately plays tricks with asthma and no self-respecting paediatric unit would deny a night's 'shared-care' to such a child.

N.B. Above, I have used the term 'β_2-adrenergic agonist'. I do not regard all members of this group of drugs as being equally safe. However, two, salbutamol and terbutaline, though there may be individual differences in response by a particular patient, are both very safe and very effective. For the sake of brevity in this, and subsequent answers, in some instances I have exampled salbutamol only.

Question 8.   Too young for salbutamol?

On the data sheet salbutamol is not advised for children under 2 years of age. There seems to be no age stated under which orciprenaline cannot be used. Confronted with a wheezy child of 6 months which, if either, of these substances would you use and in what kind of dosage? Under what circumstances would you also use antibiotics?

Salbutamol sometimes, antibiotics occasionally, orciprenaline never.

A first attack of wheezing, of short duration, in a 6-month old child could well be a respiratory syncytial virus (RSV) infection. I would teach a simple physiotherapy regime before feeds and suggest cold mist or a safely placed bowl of cold water to raise humidity. I would want to see such a baby again in 24 hours to gauge the severity of the attack, or immediately, of course, if he or she seemed to deteriorate in any way.

More severe RSV infections may require a paediatric physiotherapist to do (and teach) better percussion. I might try inhaled ipratropium through the practice nebulizer or a masked spacer (see Figure 2) but would advise a low threshold here for seeking a paediatric opinion.

The prolonged/repeatedly wheezy 6-month baby needs a different approach. Atopy, bronchial responsiveness and viral-induced mechanisms can be involved here. β_2-agonist is disappointing given orally but may work better inhaled through the nebulizer. I believe GPs prefer oral orciprenaline because a dose is given for this age group in a total mg amount in the British National Formulary (BNF) and by volume in MIMS. Salbutamol appears in a dose of mg/kg per dose in the BNF and is 'not recommended' in MIMS. There can be no other logic for preferring the old-fashioned and less specific orciprenaline. I used to give oral xanthines at this age but, because of the problem with toxicity, I no longer do so.

Inhaled ipratropium has scored better in trials at this age. A spacing device (Figure 2) gives a system with faster delivery of drugs, low expense on equipment outlay and much flexibility. Try the following in the spacer:

- Ipratropium aerosol, 2 puffs t.d.s. If no success, then:
- Salbutamol (or terbutaline) aerosol, 2 puffs q.d.s.

It is possible to add cromoglycate and/or inhaled steroid if necessary, for frequently relapsing disease.

Antibiotics inevitably creep in, especially where there is a fever, but bilateral signs in an infant with prolonged or repeated symptoms can hardly represent 'recurrent bacterial bronchopneumonia'. Physiotherapy eliminates areas of collapse from mucus plugs and reduces the fever, especially if the airway diameter is improved first with ipratropium!

However, if the GP is confronted by a 'one-off,' apparent wheezy chest infection in a previously non-wheezy child, although the infection is most likely to be viral, no harm will be done in using an antibiotic, as long as it has a broad enough spectrum, including effectiveness against both mycoplasma and chlamydia, e.g. erythromycin or ceflaclor.

Question 9.   Does croup justify a visit?

At 3 a.m. a doctor is called to see a 2-year-old with croup. The laryngeal spasm is only apparent when the child coughs or gets upset, the rest of the time there is no audible stridor. The doctor prescribes steam only. Is he correct? Could he safely have stayed in his bed and prescribed the same treatment? What proportion of simple croup turns out to be acute laryngotracheobronchitis and is this condition easy to recognize? What if the child with croup looked perfectly well but had a degree of subcostal recession?

Better to be safe than sorry. This is an unpredictable condition.

Sitting in a bathroom, alongside a bath full of hot water, with doors and windows closed usually alleviates most cases of croup.

I would always want to 'see for myself' if only to obtain a baseline of severity and exclude the rarer possibility of epiglottitis. Seeing the response to steam is reassuring. Perhaps a previously known family describing recurrent croup, a mainly allergic phenomenon, can be managed by a telephone conversation with confident parents. Acute croup is synonymous with acute laryngo-tracheitis, virtually always viral. There is a differential diagnosis for an inspiratory stridor:

- Acute epiglottitis.
- Foreign body.
- Retropharyngeal abscess.

Ninety to ninety-five per cent of acute inspiratory stridor is acute croup and although usually mild is unpredictable. An experienced GP, with competent parents, can usually see a mild case through at home.
Serious signs, indicative of epiglottitis, are:

- Dysphagia.
- Excessive salivation.
- Inability to lie flat.
- Extreme lethargy.
- Cyanosis.
- Toxic appearance.
- Neck extension.
- Suprasternal and possibly intercostal and subcostal recession, and when present, urgent (accompanied) admission (if possible forewarning the hospital) is vital.

Persistent subcostal (often combined with sternal) insuction in croup should also be monitored in hospital unless there is clear improvement in steam.

Question 10. Make space for a spacer

A doctor is called to see a temporary resident, an asthmatic 3½-year-old, who is usually treated with nebulized salbutamol. The doctor only has a spacing device and salbutamol inhaler with him. Would this be a reasonable replacement? How many 'puffs' could be safely used?

Always carry a spacing device (Figure 2). There is a high ratio of safety with salbutamol.
Spacers have repeatedly been shown to be excellent alternatives to nebulizers and many 3½-year-olds are quite expert at using

them. Only a small percentage of the drug reaches the appropriate airways and so it is safe to use many puffs (5 at least). Ensure 5–6 breaths between each puff. A peak flow whistle (supplied gratis by some pharmaceutical companies) can often be used to gauge effectiveness.

Spacers and puffs are rather imprecise. In a nebulizer we use:

- 2.5 mg salbutamol up to 3 years of age (2500 µg)
- 5.0 mg salbutamol for 3–6 years (5000 µg)
- 7.5 mg salbutamol for 6–12 years (7500 µg)

In a spacer:

- 1 puff (100 µg) – thus 5 puffs (500 µg) is still very conservative.

Question 11. Keeping your nerve with a chronic cough

A girl of 18 months has had a cough for 7 weeks which the parents insist wakes her up every night. No medicines have worked, and there are no signs of asthma. Would you suggest a paediatric opinion and/or chest X-ray?

Although it is not likely to be serious, a further opinion might be reassuring.

Night-time cough alone is an unusual manifestation of asthma at 18 months although it might be the cause. There are alternative explanations, particularly post-nasal drip in a catarrhal child or an inhaled foreign body.

I would undertake a chest X-ray if I could not find a convincing explanation. No parent is going to feel easy about such a child and I would seek such reassurance for everyone's peace of mind. There have been many cases involving inhaled foreign bodies where such an X-ray, early on, would have avoided a great deal of distress, not least for the doctors concerned.

Question 12. 'It only gets better with antibiotics'

For the fourth time in as many months an 18-month-old baby is brought to the surgery with a purulent nasal discharge, a pyrexia of 100°F, and, in spite of a clear chest, a cough. . . 'a terrible cough, Doctor. He keeps getting them. They only get better with antibiotics'. The doctor sees from the notes that the child has had

numerous courses of antibiotics from his desperate colleagues. How should he proceed?

Whatever is given at the height of an illness, before its natural resolution, is almost bound to work!

Whenever I see these children at the clinic they are, invariably, well. I instruct the mother, and my staff, that I want to see the next attack myself, straight away. Ninety per cent of times that is the last I hear of it. Usually these are children who, by reason of large families, nurseries etc., are exposed to many other children. I would tell the parents that a child of this age should be expected to get a pyrexial illness at least every 6 weeks as an essential part of the natural process of developing immunity – 'What you get now, you don't get later' – and that what is given at the height of a naturally resolving illness is almost always likely to succeed. Severe adenoidal enlargement may be present, but then symptoms would likely persist between attacks. Rare immune deficiencies often present as severe recurrent otitis, pneumonia or other life-threatening infections, and might improve with antibiotics.

One thing, however, is worth considering. If it does transpire that there is a significant bacterial infection and the GP has prescribed an antibiotic, he will be everybody's favourite. For this reason, if a positive decision is made not to give antibiotics then the child should certainly be examined with appropriate clinical care and appropriate advice given to the parents.

Question 13.   Does exercise always make asthma worse?

In spite of using β_2-agonist and steroid inhalers a child of 9 years has quite a lot of asthma while running about. Efforts are being made to overcome this with medication. In the meantime should the child be encouraged to take more exercise or less?

Properly monitored exercise should be encouraged.

It must be a prime objective for successful therapy for a child to be returned to a fully active life. Only in a tiny percentage of severe asthmatics does it become impossible to participate in some activity. Swimming of course is the likeliest salvation. There is a strong movement in Europe to use methods of 'desensitization' to exercise-induced asthma by a carefully structured training programme. The priorities should therefore be to:

• Ensure maximum compliance.
• Ensure maximum expertise is brought to bear on medication

options, especially the newer range of drugs such as nedocromil and salmeterol.
* Ensure the 'whole child' and family are evaluated to reduce 'stress factors' to a minimum.
* Ensure optimal prophylaxis against exercise-induced factors, e.g. timing of treatment, type of therapy, environmental triggers (better in warm gym than cold field).
* Start with swimming, progress to 'non-competitive', non-severely exertional exercise, e.g. walking or short jog, or gentle cycling and aerobics.
* Use a disciplined, structured, gradual programme.
* Check that there is no 'late-onset' reaction (as well as obviously watching for acute responses) especially worsening night asthma after exercise. Ensure peak flow is measured that evening.
* Ensure adequate help is available for unexpected response, e.g. a nebulizer at school; a well-informed teacher (or a school nurse); open access to practice.

Yes, encouragement always pays dividends.

Question 14. Home nebulizer – a false sense of security?

A child of 3 years has recurrent severe asthma and has been admitted to hospital on several occasions, often requiring steroids. The parents are the opposite of panicky, tending to let the situation get really bad before they call the doctor. They are very keen to try a home nebulizer. Could this end up giving them a false sense of security? Would it be better, perhaps, to give them a course of oral steroids with specific instructions on how, and when, to use them?

Education is essential. Don't leap to steroids. Consider nebulized cromoglycate.

I doubt whether nebulized β_2-agonist will make the family more at risk than they are already. You should not give up attempting to re-educate them with specific spoken and written instructions on what to record and on what to base their actions. If you have a trained asthma clinic nurse she might be of great help with this as well.

After 2.5 mg nebulized salbutamol a child should give clear signs of improvement such as:

* Having a respiratory rate of less than 50/min.
* Being able to speak clearly and slowly.
* Being able, and happy, to walk about.
* Being able to eat and drink.

Anything less of a response must be relayed to the doctor.

The question assumes that you could instruct the parents effectively on giving oral steroids. I suspect that many doctors feel safer with steroids but, personally, I still worry about opening the flood gates to steroids for children, both inhaled and oral. I would want the parents to report in before giving the steroids and be sure they have followed the more conservative lines first.

I have already mentioned that ipratropium may be more effective in this age group (see Question 8). Perhaps the best use of the nebulizer in this household would be to use it to give cromoglycate for good prophylaxis.

Question 15. Nebulized salbutamol – a deliberate overdose?

General practitioners are advised to carry nebulizers in their cars. Given that there is 25 times more salbutamol in a 2.5 mg nebule than there is in one 'puff' of inhaler, why does this not constitute an overdose? Is it common to see, in a hospital situation, overdosage of β_2-agonists?

Salbutamol has a large margin of safety.

Some children become shaky on relatively small doses of salbutamol and some become rather excitable. It is to be remembered that only a small fraction of nebulized (or puffed) drug actually reaches its destination. Remember, too, that oral salbutamol represents a high comparative dosage. All this shows how effective yet phenomenally safe this drug is. In the main it is underdosed.

Regarding the doctor carrying a nebulizer, in many cases a spacer and puffer can be just as good (see Question 10) and many doctors now use spacing devices in situations where they previously used nebulizers. They do not break down, are very easy to use and the required pressurized inhaler is usually to hand when, sometimes, the nebulizing solution is not.

Question 16. Decongestants. Comforting or calamitous?

It has always been customary to treat small children with upper respiratory infections with various decongestant substances either on the bedclothes or on the skin. There has been a suggestion that

this could have an association with cot death. Is there sufficient evidence to justify not using these comforting substances on young children?

If used they must be kept well away from the child's airway.

The conflict is 'old habits die hard' versus 'primum non nocere' ('first do no harm'). Neither the effectiveness of volatile oils as a decongestant in snuffly babies, nor their role in producing apnoea in a potentially compromised infant, is really adequately proved. Cot death phobia only heightens these battles. Some parents need 'something done' to allay their anxieties about trivial illness and force the prescription of antibiotics or symptomatic medicines, whilst others wisely accept avoidance of any doubtful medication or advice.

Thus I offer a selection of approaches in order of increasing risk:

- Tickling the nares with a teased cotton bud induces sneezing and clears the nasal passages temporarily, e.g. before feeding.
- Cold mist, or a bowl of cold water safely secreted in the child's bedroom, are harmless manoeuvres which raise humidity and improve the movement of secretions, particularly at night.
- Nose drops, 1–2 in each nostril three times per day, such as ephedrine 0.5% in saline or saline alone. This treatment should be used for a few days only and is most helpful before feeds.
- Profuse, persistent rhinorrhoea occasionally needs mechanical aspiration before feeds and in the night. A soft suction tube with bulb attachment is available in some chemists and baby shops.
- 'Vapour' products must not be put directly on a child's skin (they can burn) and must not be in a concentrated form close to the airways as reflex apnoea could occur. A small dab on old towelling several metres away from the baby will probably improve the parent's nasal perception and ease minds whilst avoiding the stated danger.
- I would consider using a small dose of antihistamine/sympathomimetic decongestant in a child of 2 years. I favour Dimotapp paediatric elixir 2.5 ml b.d. at this stage. Brompheniramine does not produce hallucinations like some similar, commonly used preparations (even those earmarked as suitable for children). Promethazine elixir 5 mg/ml is available across the counter and 5 ml b.d. may be tried in a younger child (i.e. 0.5 mg/kg per dose for the average 10 kg, 1-year-old). Occasionally it produces irritability and paradoxical sleeplessness, not dangerous, but not applauded by the majority of parents.

Question 17. Think twice, or at least once, before using steroids

How would you reassure your endocrinologist colleague that the inhaled steroid you are considering prescribing for his 4-year-old son, cromoglycate not having worked, will cause no harm?

I would not reassure. I would discuss the advantages and disadvantages of the treatment available.

Just two words of caution. Check compliance. Cromoglycate is rather bitter tasting and it requires experimentation with delivery to ensure the child is truly unresponsive rather than non-compliant. I have mentioned before (Question 14) that it can be given by nebulizer.

For a child of this age with mild asthma I would prefer to maximize β_2-agonist therapy by using, perhaps, a slow release form e.g. Volmax which children > 3 years can often swallow, or a long-acting form e.g. salmeterol given as a metered dose inhaler (MDI) through a spacing device.

At the present time, the international concensus group would encourage GPs to have a specialist take the first step into steroids. The drugs do, indeed, suppress the adrenals if the dosage exceeds $400 \, \mu g/m^2/day$ of beclomethasone, for example, and nobody yet knows for sure what will be the effects of much lower doses over a very long period.

However, if the asthma warrants inhaled steroids they should not be withheld and can be very beneficial. It is a balance of pros and cons. I would not be parental to my colleague and I would share the facts. If everything else has been tried methodically, steroids in small doses would be a justifiable recommendation.

Throat, nose and ear

Question 18. Could it be epiglottitis?

A child of 6 years complains of a very sore throat. He seems unable even to swallow his own saliva. He has a history of tonsillitis in the past but the doctor is concerned lest this be epiglottitis. Is it reasonable for the doctor to hospitalize the child without examining his throat?

My first thoughts in this case would be a quinsy rather than epiglottitis. A peritonsillar abscess occurs as a complication of severe tonsillitis and produces severe pain and dysphagia. Epiglottitis, virtually always a *Haemophilus influenzae* infection, is said to be rare beyond 5 years, though my GP colleague assures me that in his experience he has seen as many adult cases as children (an observation also made at the local district general hospital – there must be something about the Thames Valley air!)

Epiglottitis would be more likely to produce stridor and hoarseness as well as dysphagia and the other signs described earlier (see Question 9). Nevertheless, if epiglottitis is in any way suspected DO NOT TRY AND EXAMINE THE THROAT BY DEPRESSING THE TONGUE. The toxic child could drop down dead in front of you with ventricular fibrillation or be projected into an acute respiratory obstruction. This would be the clinical equivalent of doing a vaginal examination, at home, on a pregnant woman bleeding at 32 weeks. In any event, in this case, if the alternative diagnosis is likely to be quinsy, and particularly if the mother says the attack is worse than, or different to, any of the others, you are going to send the child into hospital come what may and it can be argued that you need not take the risk of looking at the throat at all. If epiglottitis is suspected, accompany the child in the ambulance. GPs should always carry a medicut or tracheal trocar to attempt an emergency airway if all else fails.

Question 19. Tonsillitis. Medical or surgical problem?

A child of 2½ years is brought to the doctor hot, unwell and vomiting. On examination the tonsils are found to be covered with exudate. Reference to the notes shows this to be the fourth such attack in 6 months. What action should the doctor take? If

referral is advised should it be to the ENT department or the paediatrician?

Medical treatment is generally preferable to surgery but surgery is better in given situations.

Recurrent tonsillitis caused by haemolytic streptococcus A in children is quite common. After appropriate treatment the streptococcus disappears from throat swabs but comes back with the next attack (the recurrent group). With some children the streptococcus continues, in lesser quantities, to be present all the time (the relapsing group). These children sometimes need intramuscular penicillin and oral rifampicin to get them out of the carrier state.

Tonsillectomy has to be considered a risky operation that makes ear, nose and throat surgeons understandably cautious. Nevertheless, in partnership with large adenoids, upper airway obstruction, particularly during sleep or if it makes eating very difficult, is a clear indication for surgical action and I have seen such surgery carried out, justifiably, on infants as young as 9 months.

Recurrent quinsy (peritonsillar abcess) is always an indication for tonsillectomy.

Question 20.   Sore throat – night cramps

A boy of 7 years complains of waking in the night with cramping pains in the legs. These attacks usually occur when he has a cold or a sore throat. Is there any cause for concern? Have they anything to do with 'growing pains'?

There is probably nothing much wrong.

If the pains are bilateral, cramp-like, located in muscles especially calf, then the description is fairly typical of 'night cramp' and may occur after an energetic day or appear around the time of an upper respiratory tract infection in the 4–8 year age group.

Are these the same as the 'growing pains' of an older age group (8–12-year-olds) whose pain can occur in the day as well as at night, often sited around the knee, shin or ankle? I see these particularly in thin Asian children.

• As with recurrent abdominal pain, meticulous history and examination at presentation is an essential reassurance for parent (and doctor), for although I believe many have a psychosomatic origin, I rarely pinpoint a convincing dynamic.

- Hyperlaxity of joints; chilblains (beware child abuse); and the juvenile osteochondritis syndromes may indicate different causes.
- A short history and severe pain always frightens me into seeking a blood film to exclude leukaemia. Severe pain in one site in a bony area calls for an X-ray or bone scan, e.g. an osteoid osteoma or worse.
- Rheumatic fever is increasing again, but without a full Duckett–Jones assembly of criteria you should not seriously confuse a direct cause and effect between tonsillitis and limb pains.

Question 21. Snotty nosed kid

A consultant paediatrician finds that one of his own children, aged 4 years, has a permanently snotty nose. Should he ignore this or should he, for the sake of his own public image, be tempted to treat it in some way? And if so, with what?

A handkerchief!

Being an insightful paediatrician I suppose I must assume this is the first time since birth that the offending doctor has been home, i.e. this is a typical catarrhal child. Onset at 4 years would be uncommon and perhaps only 'allergy' a likely explanation. The protracted catarrhal child has been best understood thanks to a GP (Dr John Fry) rather than any card-carrying paediatrician. You must avoid missing:

- Bilateral/unilateral foreign bodies.
- Marked septal deviation.
- Massive mucosal swelling of severe allergy.
- Polyps (in unsuspected cystic fibrosis).
- The mouth-breathing, dry-tongued, night-snoring and waking, poor hearing and indistinct speaking of severe adenoidal hyperplasia which, amazingly, still slips past everyone's attention.

All of the above have very specific remedies.

- Infections with bacteria and viruses.

Mild responses to house-dust mite and other allergens and mild immunodevelopmental delay are factors accounting for the vast majority or other prolonged or persistent rhinitis and, to be honest, nothing really alters the course for these very inconvenienced children and their families. Decongestants, antihistamines, mast cell stabilizers and topical corticosteroids are all over-used and over-praised. 'Doing no harm' applies here when I

remind readers of the many children that have daytime hallucinations or night time terrors as a result of some 'decongestant'
preparations, not just mistaken adult doses or preparations but
some specifically directed at children.

Teaching a 4-year-old how to use a handkerchief (or tissue)
without Valsalva effect (i.e. wiping, not blowing) is probably the
best way to spend your consultation.

Question 22. Secretory otitis. Surgical or medical problem?

**The mother of a 3-year-old child is concerned because the health
visitor says her child is somewhat deaf. There is a history of otitis
media and the GP diagnoses secretory otitis. When he suggests a
consultation with an ENT surgeon the mother is most anxious that
the child should not have grommets inserted because her neigh-
bour's child, having had the same operation at the same age,
developed quite severe infection. Might a paediatrician's opinion
at this age be different to that of an ENT surgeon?**

It might. The pendulum may be swinging back to the medical
(conservative) approach.

A recently published analysis (Figure 3) sets the background to
the obvious dilemma surrounding opinions on how to handle 'glue
ear'. The surgical warfare waged on tympanic membranes is now
being submitted to harsh scrutiny by all those involved, particularly ear, nose and throat (ENT) surgeons themselves. There is a
limitless call on procedures no one can agree over, for a disease
no one is sure has meaningful existence:

- Is the diagnosis one of symptoms, e.g. deafness, pain, recurring
  infection, speech and language delay with clear clinical criteria
  on auroscopy, or mobility responses or tympanometry or
  audiometry or a combination of some or all of these? Does it
  require proof of fluid present by aspiration?
- Is medical management sufficiently evaluated and consistently
  applied to delineate surgical alternatives?
- Are surgeons adequately informed of all important morbidity
  events to evaluate short-term gain against long-term conse-
  quences?

For the record, my opinion would recommend surgical opinion if:

- Recurrent otitis media occurred unremittingly every month for
  6 months when most of the usual criteria for glue ear, i.e.
  auroscopic 'glue', poor mobility or tympanometric equivalent,

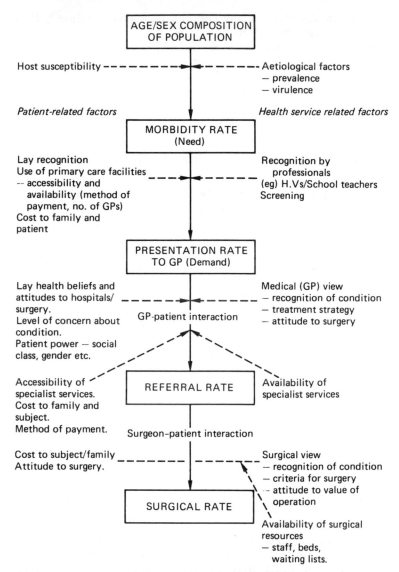

Figure 3 Determinants of a surgical rate (in the UK). Black N.A. (1985) in *Progress in Child Health* (J.A. Macfarlane ed.), Vol. 2, p. 169, Edinburgh: Churchill Livingstone

significant hearing loss (>20 dB in the better ear) were still present between attacks (preferably assessed at least 3 weeks after the last episode). These would have to persist despite a long-term trial (6–12 weeks) of prophylactic antibiotics (cotrimoxazole) and decongestant to buy a suitable period of 'respite' healing.

• Other associated factors would cause greater anxiety such as poor speech and language development in a child of this age (or younger). The impact of repeated, intermittent disruption of hearing seems greater on those acquiring expressive speech than those in which it has developed. (NB Most surgery was performed on 5–7-year-olds in an Oxford study in 1975–1980.)

• I am grateful to work alongside gracious, surgically conservative, child-orientated and self-critical ENT surgical colleagues. In this harmonious setting we can share opinions, understand respective criteria and thus present parents with both opinions discussed to consensus. I would counsel as conservative an approach as I could possibly muster until better audit and research illuminates the disappointing darkness of our current understanding.

Question 23. Hay fever in a toddler

In May a child of 3½ years is brought to the doctor with a profusely running nose, red eyes and a slight wheeze. The mother feels sure that the child has hay fever as she has it herself. Is such a diagnosis reasonable at this age? From what age on would you make the diagnosis?

Hay fever is common in children under 5 years and it is particularly recognized by parents with hay fever.

Mothers are always correct in their observations and more often than not in their deductions. That is my genuine belief and experience. Anyone who suffers from hay fever can recognize it in their children. Allergic rhinitis is incredibly common in young children (under 5s), leading to persistent nasal congestion (snuffles) with or without mucoid discharge, mouth breathing, cough on first lying down and on waking, producing 'rattles' often confused with wheeze, and snoring through the night. This differs from the more persistent cough throughout the night or sudden onset of cough in the early hours leading often to waking and retching, more suggestive of lower airway involvement i.e. asthma.

Hay fever is after all only seasonal allergic rhinitis. Mothers would easily recognize an exacerbation of symptoms in May to July, especially if associated with streaming, irritating often suffused eyes; sneezing and profuse increase of clear mucoid nasal secretions and particularly if these symptoms had appeared at a similar time in a previous year.

It is not a diagnosis I would make in the first year of life.

Question 24. Blocked nose and infant feeding

An infant of 10 days is having difficulty in breast feeding because of a blocked nose. Are nose drops contraindicated at such a young age? If so, what is the alternative? If not, which ones are best used?

Only use nose drops if absolutely necessary. Normal saline first and, if that doesn't work, ephedrine 0.5%.

Intermittent nasal mucus (snuffles) is almost invariable in the newborn, probably resulting from a combination of effects:

* The neonate is an obligate nose-breather and snorts his way past any secretions.
* The nasal passages are anatomically small.
* The nasal mucosa swells and has generous mucus secreting glands responding to the physical assault and bombardment with foreign particles as sharp contrast to its protected sterile bathing of intra-uterine life. Cold air, dust, pollens and cigarette smoke are almost unavoidable.

It is important to consider other, admittedly rare, causes if the blocked nose is severe, persistent, non-mucoid or unilateral:

* Marked septal deviation.
* Acute viral, bacterial or even protozoal (syphilis) infections.
* Perhaps true 'allergic rhinitis'.
* Congenital anomalies, e.g. haemangioma; partial or complete choanal atresia.
* Drug-withdrawal syndromes, e.g. from heroin-addicted mothers.
* Mucopolysaccharidoses.

Most 'physiological' cases require no treatment. It may be necessary, however, in order to help feeding, to use some of the remedies already mentioned in Question 16 but which, in this context, I touch on again.

* Posturing the infant prone and slightly head-down before feeds for a few minutes may gravitate secretions out of mischief.
* A 'teased' cotton-bud gently wiped inside the external nares often induces sneezing and precipitates what the infant so frequently does spontaneously at this age, to clear his/her airways.
* An occasional drop of normal saline, especially before meals, will clear mucus or precipitate a sneeze. If used frequently maceration of nasal skin may occur.
* Ephedrine 0.5% in saline if used for more than a few days in continuity is likely to precipitate a 'rebound' mucosal congestion and relapse or even worsen the situation. Avoid if possible.

- A mechanical suction bulb, sterilized with the bottles, may be needed to aspirate excessive secretions, again often prior to feeds.
- Increasing room humidity, if necessary with a cold mist humidifier, is favoured by many (including me), but frowned on by academics as promoting 'allergen' production.

Have I sat on the fence? I'm a reluctant nose-drop user at this age, with saline (0.9%) as my first line and ephedrine 0.5% in saline my fall-back agent, but both of these very conservatively applied.

Infections

Question 25. How long off school?

How long would you keep a child off school with otitis media? With tonsillitis? How soon after the attacks would you allow a return to such activities as swimming or playing football?

I have no rules about withholding from school.

I would mostly trust parents but try to rationalize for them a few good reasons to delay return – mostly obvious, e.g. high fever, vomiting, considerable pain and marked lethargy. Streptococcus A in the throat is infectious but that is rarely identified. Good schools cope with midday antibiotics (modern antibiotics and preparations may often avoid the need for these).

Hopefully schools will also be prepared to co-operate with parents and accept 'no competitive sport' for a few days until the child is back to full zest.

Regarding swimming, one acute attack of otitis media deserves 2 weeks repair time, and no diving for 4 weeks. In the case of a number of close attacks of otitis media I would advise a term off swimming – or a change of swimming pools. With regard to swimming and ear problems generally it is not always realized, by parents, that most of the problems are caused by blockage of the eustachian tubes following nasal congestion brought on by the chemicals in the swimming pool water. It does not therefore protect the vulnerable child to give him ear plugs. Better a nose clip!

Question 26. Perilous purpura

A boy of 3 years has been unwell for 2 days. The mother has brought him to the doctor's early evening surgery and pointed to the purpuric spots that have appeared upon the abdomen within the past 4 hours. The child does not appear particularly ill. Can the doctor safely leave the child until the next morning when he hopes that a blood test will exclude a blood dyscrasia thus pointing to a diagnosis of Henoch–Schonlein or could he be missing a diagnosis of meningococcal meningitis?

Think and move urgently!

- Purpura and peril live hand in hand and there is no point in procrastination.

- Purpura appearing in a perfectly well child, without enlarged lymph nodes or splenomegaly, 7–10 days after an acute illness like chicken-pox is likely to be due to 'idiopathic thrombocytopenia'.
- Colicky abdominal pain, with bloody diarrhoea, pains in large joints especially knees and a classic distribution of purpura (with or without other skin lesions, e.g. urticarial, erythematous) on extensor surfaces of the arms, legs and buttocks – but *not* on the trunk or face – can be confidently classified as 'anaphylactoid purpura' (Henoch–Schonlein).
  Both these conditions warrant hospital assessment anyway, but remove immediacy.
- Where **any doubt** exists the child must be sent (preferably taken) urgently to the nearest paediatric unit. Systemic penicillin (IM or IV) if immediately available, should be given, even if the child seems well.
- Remember that some children with septicaemia or meningitis only begin to look ill very shortly before they are very ill indeed, if not terminal.
- Research is rapidly changing initial management of meningococcal disease and I predict we will soon be giving dexamethasone shortly before cefotaxime – but these drugs need to be immediately available and be given systemically.

Question 27.   Antibiotics without diagnosis

In the past it was the habit of many doctors when faced with a small child with a pyrexia, to prescribe a course of antibiotics even though no focal cause for the infection could be found. With the growing awareness that a high proportion of these infections are viral this practice has been widely criticized and, particularly by younger doctors, been largely abandoned in this zeal to practise 'good medicine'. Is it possible that fewer children with covert, possibly hazardous bacterial infections such as pyelonephritis, are being treated than previously? Under what circumstances, if any, would you give antibiotics 'blind'?

'Blind' antibiotics can be more hazardous than none at all.

Over 90% of childhood infections are non-bacterial and even those which are, rarely warrant 'blind therapy'. I would want to differentiate what might be called 'strategic therapy'. This comprises:

- Clinical localization of site of infection, e.g. ears, lower respiratory tract, superficial wound, etc.

- Knowledge of likely infecting (bacterial) agents in that site.
- Knowledge of influence of age on likely infecting agent.
- Knowledge of current sensitivities of such agents *in your community* to the useful (i.e. mainly oral) antibiotics.
- Knowledge of antibiotic preparations, side effects, dosages, tolerance, and cost.

Although there is considerable discussion about the need for antibiotics in, say, acute otitis media, in such a situation the use of antibiotics is at least considerably narrowed and rationalized.

However, the sequel to an ill-diagnosed and treated urinary tract infection is years of follow-up and investigation, at great cost to the child, the family and the health service. I use the word cost in its broadest sense not specifically in financial terms. It is therefore hard to justify blind therapy in suspected urinary tract infection; similarly, for cases of pyrexia of unknown origin and upper respiratory illness except, as indicated, severe acute otitis. If you are able, it would be wiser to contract with your local paediatric provider to ensure a supra-pubic aspiration – not so difficult these days with ultrasound help – on a sick, febrile infant, plus a blood culture or a chest X-ray whenever you need one (24 hour service). Not everyone enjoys these privileges, however so:

- In a sick, febrile infant (under 1 year) try to obtain an adequate urine (within 1–2 hours) and start antibiotics trimethoprim 4–8 mg/kg per day before the culture is available if microscopy shows organisms.
- If purpura appears – see Question 20 – give systemic (IM/IV) penicillin *without delaying admission*. Cefotaxime (Claforan) in a 500 mg vial – 25 mg/kg as an initial dose, IM/IV – will soon be recommended as well as or instead of penicillin.
- A sick febrile infant with lower respiratory signs should be given erythromycin 25–50 mg/kg per day or cephalexin 25–50 mg/kg per day (each divided into four doses) unless you confidently diagnose viral bronchiolitis.

Question 28.   Whooping cough contacts

None of the children aged 4, 3, 2 years and 6 months in a family of epileptic parents have had whooping cough vaccination. The child of 4 years contracts an upper respiratory tract infection at nursery school which later turns out to be whooping cough. The doctor sees the family and notes that the children of 3 years and 6 months have developed a coryzal type illness. How should the doctor proceed?

Treat the baby.

Although given more in hope than conviction, erythromycin has claimants for its modifying the severity of an attack, and it does sterilize the respiratory tract very quickly so reducing infectivity. A total of 25–50 mg/kg per day divided into four doses for 7–10 days should *certainly* be given to the infant. If the baby develops severe paroxysms salbutamol 0.1 mg/kg 6-hourly, orally, may help. You should not hesitate to admit the infant for tube-feeding, physiotherapy and shared nursing care if the disease looks at all severe.

Question 29.   Always investigate childhood UTI

After how many attacks of urinary tract infection (UTI) would you investigate a girl of 6 years? A boy of the same age?

Investigate after ONE attack – boys and girls.

The golden rule, preached by paediatricians for years, now cast in tablets of stone by a working group of the Royal College of Physicians research unit (January 1991) – including two GPs and a lay parent – is that all children diagnosed as having urinary tract infection should have some form of imaging after the first proved infection.

Children who presented 30 years ago with a UTI now have a 20% risk of hypertension and a 10% risk of chronic renal failure.

Question 30.   Recurrent vaginal discharge. Abuse or not?

A little girl of 18 months is brought to the doctor with vaginal discharge. There is slight excoriation but no real evidence of any physical injury or abuse. This is the third occasion that the child has had this problem. Previously a *Strep. faecalis* had been grown on culture and the condition resolved on amoxycillin. At what stage should the child be investigated, and how? Are there any subtle signs that might easily be missed by the child's family doctor that might lead you to a consideration of child sexual abuse?

If in any doubt refer to an expert in these matters. It is most likely not to be the result of sexual abuse but it probably needs a specialist opinion to say so.

It is vital to be confident and competent about the physical examination. It is just as important to check that:

- The child has not had frequent antibiotics for other reasons, as these alter the perineal microflora and especially promote fungal infection.
- There are no threadworms present.
- No bubble baths or 'designer additives' are used in the bath water.
- 'Personal hygiene' is adequate, e.g. nappy changes frequent enough, wiping is from 'front to back'.
- Chemical wipes are avoided.

These may all tip the balance towards considering recurrent low grade infection, chemical or allergic dermatitis as the most likely explanation. Frequently I find inflammation (dermatitis) of the surrounding perivulval and perianal skin and there are conditions such as contact eczema, lichen sclerosus et atrophicus and psoriasis that need to be recognized.

Examining the genitalia needs a lot of training and experience regarding normal and abnormal appearances. If you cannot see all the details shown in Figure 4, you cannot be certain of the diagnosis and your technique will be inadequate. Your database

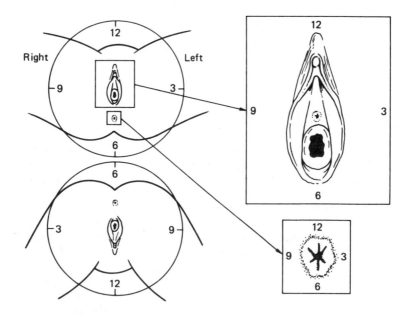

Figure 4 'Clockface' orientation diagram for female child's genitalia

of normality is then going to be suspect. If any doubt exists at all, ask a consultant to help.

- Do not confront parents or children with leading or difficult questions.
- Do not feed unsubstantiated 'anxieties' onwards.
- Do know which local paediatricians are experienced in sexual abuse matters. You should always have knowledge of the Child Protection Team in your area.
- Do talk directly to the consultant if at all possible.
- Ensure you find a stimulating, well-run child abuse course to go on sometime soon.

Most paediatricians I know will see chronic or recurrent vaginal discharge these days almost as fast as suspected meningitis.

If you have any suspicion of abuse and the appearance of the child's genitalia deviates from the norm, a copy of Figure 4 with 'clock-face' orientation can be used to note any abnormality.

Question 31. 'He keeps getting a temperature, Doctor'

For a period of some weeks an apparently healthy toddler of 2 years is grizzly for about 1 day in 4 or 5. On each occasion the mother takes the child's temperature and finds it to be 100°F or more. She gives the child paracetamol and he is well – and apyrexial – the next day. What is the most likely diagnosis? Can a child become pyrexial in ordinary circumstances simply by being too hot?

Though the cause is not likely to be serious, I would be happier to do a few investigations.

The only simple explanations are:

- A string of unrelated mild infections, usually upper respiratory, and seen in the younger siblings of large families or when a toddler enters a day nursery or shares a child-minder with other tots.
- The hidden enemy – relapsing or unresolving occult urinary tract disease.
- An infectious disease with a prolonged prodroma such as incipient mumps or chicken pox.

It is certainly possible to overdress and overheat infants and toddlers. I'm afraid the story would goad me into doing:

- A blood culture (combined with blood film).
- A throat swab (looking for Group A streptococcus).

- A Mantoux 1 in 1000 to exclude TB.
- A urine culture.
- Probably a chest X-ray (e.g. Mycoplasma pneumonia can be fairly inconspicuous and prolonged),

if I could not pinpoint an explanation clinically.

Question 32.   What constitutes a meningococcal 'close contact'?

A doctor is besieged by a horde of mothers whose children have been 'in contact' with a case of meningococcal meningitis. He is told by the powers that be that only close contacts require rifampicin. How close is close? What about the doctor who examined the screaming child's throat? Does rifampicin itself cause any problems?

It depends on the age and the community involved. Rifampicin rarely causes any problems except by interaction with other drugs.

We are all afraid of the unknown, especially an unknown with a lethal or spiteful reputation. It is very probable that the virulence of the meningococcus is determined more by extraneous circumstances than inherent in the bacterium itself. A concomitant viral illness may lower host immunity or act as a 'phage' vector for the meningococcus. Age, nutritional, social, hygiene and stress factors may also have equal or greater importance.

There is, however, an undeniable increased risk of infection in close contacts, remembering that the overall risk in the UK is still very small.

Closeness will always be defined by guidelines and individual risks must still be weighed by a skilled clinician. Thus:

- The attack rate is particularly high in the under 4s.
- This age-group attends playgroups and nurseries – a vulnerable group with prolonged contact. All attending children and staff must be urgently contacted, examined, swabbed (oropharyngeal) and started on chemoprophylaxis.
- Eating, living and sleeping in the same household for 4 hours or more in the 7 days prior to the onset of disease in the index case constitutes undoubted 'close contact'. All such cases, usually just the family, are seen as soon as possible, examined, swabbed and given chemoprophylaxis. Neighbours and kissing contacts will have to be assessed individually if they come close to these descriptions.

- School contacts are not so straightforward. If a single case only, all *classmates* may be swabbed. Carrier rates of 10% or less can be handled by just treating positive carriers. A rate higher than 10% may push doctors to give all classmates (and staff) chemoprophylaxis. With high carrier rates surveillance of carrier status in their respective households may need to be pursued.

A situation of two or more cases in the same class should lead to examination, swabbing and chemoprophylaxis of all classmates ahead of results. Carriers identified will lead to further surveillance of their family.

Doctors and health workers are not a very vulnerable group statistically – at least from infection as a result of index case contact. However, it would be reasonable to suggest that:

- Mouth to mouth resuscitation of the index case;
- Suction by oral tube device (no longer a recommended technique anyway) of secretions of the index case;
- Being spat at or coughed explosively at from close range by the index case;

might be circumstances in which the health worker has a swab taken and starts chemoprophylaxis.

Just to remind readers that the dosage of rifampicin for chemoprophylaxis is

5 mg/kg b.d. for 2 days for infants under 12 months
10 mg/kg b.d. for 2 days from 12 months to 12 years
600 mg b.d. for 2 days thereafter

For this short period of time rifampicin is remarkably free of problems, but it must be remembered that:

- It colours urine red and unless forewarned parents and patients may be horrified. Contact lenses should not be affected in this sort of time span.
- A rare patient could develop hypersensitivity response with severe hepatic inflammation, but I have not seen or heard of that in my lifetime on a 2-day course.
- It is a powerful enzyme inducer and you must know what other drugs the patient is on as the chemoprophylaxis can negate the effects, e.g. theophylline, anticonvulsants, or the contraceptive pill.

Question 33. Painful hip. A diagnostic dilemma

A boy of 4 years complains of pains in the knee. He is limping and has an upper respiratory tract infection (URTI). Examination

shows him to have a painful restriction in the movement of his
right hip. The GP diagnoses 'irritable hip syndrome'. The paediatrician agrees with this diagnosis. For how long should the boy
rest? Is the condition sometimes recurrent, particularly with
further URTI?

I would advise bed rest at home for a few days but if there is any
pyrexia the child should be in hospital.

If he were febrile I would admit him to hospital where I would
hope he would have a blood culture, full blood count, ESR, viral
serology, X-rays and an ultrasound, possibly a needle aspiration
if there were any effusion. I would anticipate that he would be
put on intravenous antibiotics whilst awaiting the result of these
tests.

Recurrent pain in the hip does occur, and, as always, may be
referred, e.g. from spine, pelvis and knee or due to to disease *in
situ*. I would always want to exclude underlying serious pathology
and never assume such symptoms were 'innocent':

• Hyperlaxity syndrome – not uncommon, liable to repeated
  minor trauma.
• Chronic low-grade infection, e.g. brucella, typhoid, even staphy-
  lococcal abscesses in spine. Mycobacteria (TB) in spine or hip.
• Osteochondritis of spine (Scheuermann's) or hip (Perthes)
  occasionally present early.
• Pauciarticular juvenile arthritis affecting knee/hip.
• Bony secondaries, e.g. from neuroblastoma/leukaemia.

Bone scans, although not infallible, are proving more informative (and with less irradiation) than X-rays as an initial investigation.

Development

Question 34. Going metric

A doctor used to pounds and ounces is confused by the metric system. Is there a rapid use table for the average child that will make life easier?

Yes. See Table 3.

Question 35. When is little, too little?

A small child is, in the view of some, not considered to be thriving if he or she is under the tenth percentile. When would you investigate a child under this figure? When would you consider it not necessary to investigate a child below the third percentile?

Consistent rate of growth is far more important than any one measurement.

No single measurement defines anything. Weight is particularly misleading as the daily variation in bodyweight in a child (drink, evacuation, etc.) is as wide as the actual accumulated weight over 6 months. The ability to accurately measure height in children (and adults) requires the same assessor, using a checkable measure, with a consistent methodology (5 minutes good training) – and equipment costing as little as £50 (see Figure 5). It is important to understand a few basic 'average' concepts:

- One third of a child's growth (20" or 50 cm) occurs before birth and if you are born very small you are going to show up as small in the subsequent components.
- Another 10" (25 cm) of growth occurs in the 1st year. A total of 30" (75 cm) constitutes the infant component of growth heavily influenced by nutritional factors.
- The next (childhood) component through 1–11 years adds about 27½" (70 cm) and depends largely on growth hormone. Smaller persons travel in smaller increments than large ones, but there should be a consistent rate of growth suitable for whichever track you are stuck in (see the *velocity* chart, Figure 5). Falling outside that (below 25th or above 75th of velocity) over 6–12 months means you need shunting to the experts.

Table 3. Rapid use table

Age:	Birth	5/12	1yr	2	3	4	5	6	7	8	9	10	11
Simple Simon	Birth weight in pounds (BW)	BW×2	BW×3	BW×4	Now add 5 pounds for each year of age								
Weight (pounds) 50th percentile	7	14	21	28	33	38	43	48	53	58	63	68 (⅔adult)	
European (Rounded up to 0.5 kg)	3	6	9½	13	15	17.5	19.5	22	24	26.5	28.5	30	
Height (inches) 50th percentile	20		30			40		45		50			55
Height (cm)	51		76			102		114		127			140
Rounded up Think! (cm)	50					100				125			
Surface area (m^2) approx. (adult = 1.73)	0.2		0.5			0.75				1.0			
Peak flow litres minute 50th percentile Normal allows ± 15%						100 (85–115)	150 (130–170)	200 (170–230)		250 (210–290)		300 (255–345)	

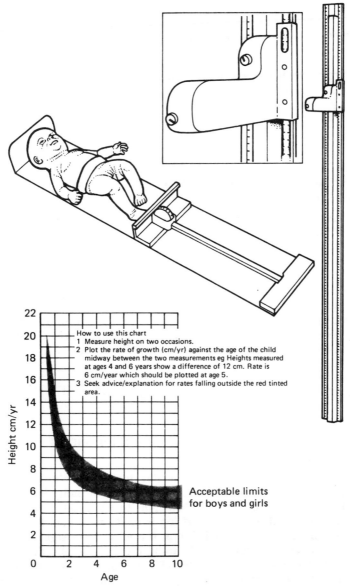

How to use this chart
1 Measure height on two occasions.
2 Plot the rate of growth (cm/yr) against the age of the child midway between the two measurements eg Heights measured at ages 4 and 6 years show a difference of 12 cm. Rate is 6 cm/year which should be plotted at age 5.
3 Seek advice/explanation for rates falling outside the red tinted area.

Acceptable limits for boys and girls

Figure 5 Height measuring equipment. Full chart available from Castlemead Publications, Welwyn Garden City

- Finally, the sex steroids determine the pubertal component. This starts earlier (average 11 years old) in girls and takes them from 55" (140 cm) to 64" (162 cm).

- Boys start later (average 13 years old) but travel further from 59" (150 cm) to 69" (175 cm).
- Do not forget that genes mainly determine end points and the mid-parental height (preferably measured) should be noted.

Armed with this knowledge, a good history and examination and 2 good recordings over a 6-month period (don't forget head circumference too) you should have no difficulties.

Question 36.   One musculoskeletal defect – keep on looking

It is said that finding one musculoskeletal abnormality in a child should lead you to look for others. Does this rule generally apply?

Yes.
Extrinsic or deforming factors acting on normal or malformed tissues can produce a large variety of fetal pathologies. The simplest example is the above-average incidence of congenital hip dislocation (CDH) in cases of extended breech presentation. Five per cent of children with significant talipes also have CDH. It is always worth looking harder if you have any reason to be suspicious.

Question 37.   Hip or miss? The dilemma of congenital dislocation

A child is examined at a 6-week developmental check and the doctor can find no hip click nor see any abnormality in the skin creases. At 10 months the child begins to walk, develops a limp and a congenital dislocation of hip is confirmed. Has the doctor necessarily missed the condition at 6 weeks? How significant are asymmetrical skin creases and should they, in the absence of any other abnormality, lead to referral? Can hips become dislocated during early childhood? Can hips be dislocated by over-enthusiastic examination?

Hip examination is not Holy Writ. It is often unnecessary, untimely and, if carried out inexpertly, frankly dangerous.
After years of screening for CDH we have all become frustrated at the persistent failures. Some are due to inexperienced screeners,

with poor technique, doing the wrong test at an inappropriate time – at 6 weeks for example! Now, however, extensive use of ultra-· sound has helped us understand that even in the best hands some hips are destined to dislocate even when they are found and treated early. We believe these cases are due to dysplastic – ill developed – acetabulae that fail to develop or improve with time or treatment. Some of these hips may, indeed, be in place after birth only to slip out later.

It is also true that over-enthusiastic screening is dangerous with the risk of avascular necrosis being greater when an intact hip is dislocated.

It is best to examine later than 48 hours after birth and before 7 days. Only experienced (trained) persons should test the hips and there must be a focus on real high-risk situations:

- A family history of congenital dislocation of the hips.
- An extended breech delivery.
- The presence of other musculo-skeletal abnormalities, e.g. talipes.

I believe a clearly defined strategy is long overdue to diminish the number of hip tests and each examination should be recorded on a personal child health record giving audit potential.

With regard to skin creases and their significance, I do not think I have ever found them significant at all. Certainly I cannot remember making a diagnosis of CDH on 'abnormal' skin creases, alone, that was confirmed by further investigation.

Question 38. Can he see and hear?

An anxious mother bringing her child for a 6-week developmental check-up says that there is both deafness and myopia in the family and she is worried that the child's hearing or sight may be faulty. At what stage can you reassure her that all is well? How much REAL idea can you get at 6 weeks?

Gross defects in seeing and hearing should certainly show themselves by 6 weeks.

In a case like this the mother's observations and worries are of considerable significance.

Ask:

- Does the baby stop sucking at an unexpected loud sound such as a dog bark or a sibling cry?
- Does the baby startle to a loud noise such as a door slam or hand clap, by blinking, dilating pupils or opening shut eyes?

- Does the baby quieten his mild cries or freeze his movements at the soft call of the out-of-view parent?
- Does the baby smile or show interest at the face of the parent without adjuvant sound and follow their movements?

These are now proved good indicators of adequately developing sight and hearing. It is usually easy at 6 weeks to check and demonstrate that the pupils react to light directly and consensually, that there is no squint, that the media are clear (red reflex· from the ophthalmoscope light on the baby's fundus in a darkened room), and that the baby will follow your face as you move across the horizontal visual plane.

- Pick up the baby and hold him vertically, facing you, with his head just above yours and rotate yourself on the spot. Rotatory nystagmus, first in one direction and then the other, seen occurring in the baby indicates that a seeing infant is fixing on his surroundings.
- Hearing is more difficult to demonstrate convincingly to the parent (and oneself) but a slightly fussing baby will freeze movement or dilate pupils, or stop crying to the mother's soft call or the slight ring of an out of sight hand bell.

You can reassure most times, but if no positive test occurs, I would not hesitate to refer to the relevant expert (with the associated technology, computerized sensors, acoustic EEG, VERs, etc.) for early assessment.

Question 39. Birth, bonding and the anaesthetized mother

A woman has a Caesarian section under a general anaesthetic. She becomes very agitated that this period of unconsciousness might have interfered with the instant 'at birth' bonding with the baby. Has she any justification for this anxiety?

No.
    Life can be full of disappointments and some people set themselves up for a serious fall. I do not believe that bonding is a 'South Pacific', 'One Enchanted Evening' only, experience. It takes time, a long time, and I hope that professionals have now learned how to help rather than hinder the process.
    Anyway, couldn't father video the whole affair?

Question 40. The yo-yo testicle

Irate parents come to the surgery saying that they have been told that their 4-year-old child needs an operation for an undescended right testicle, though the doctor who had done the 6-week developmental check reassured them that both testes were in the scrotum. Could the doctor have been correct in that assertion? At what age should a child with undescended testicles be referred?

'In the scrotum' is not the same as 'fully descended'.

Testes are best verified as descended at birth, provided that the examiner is satisfied that they can be pulled completely to the bottom of the scrotum.

This needs to be accurately recorded, as fully descended testes do not change their minds later. Cremasteric muscle development makes retractability increasingly more powerful after the age of 1 year.

If the testis is not fully descended by 3 months, an interested surgeon (with a special interest in paediatrics) should be asked to see the infant in order to plan surgery at an optimal time. Specialized paediatric surgeons may do this for those aged under 1 year, but most choose 15–18 months.

Question 41. Lumpy breasts

At various ages, particularly in early infancy and during puberty, children can develop mastitis. Are there any circumstances in which you would regard, with concern, lumps in a child's breast?

Yes.

Lumps are really unusual and if you do not recognize a disc-like enlargement, often slightly tender or sensitive, of breast tissue directly under the nipple, send forth hastily. Breast enlargement that appears for the first time beyond the neonatal period (one month) and before the pubertal period (under 8 years) is premature thelarche. Although mostly benign (seen in girls only) and due to small surges of oestrogens released from ovarian follicles they do need careful reviewing, and at least an ultrasound view of the ovaries (and uterus). I would leave it to an interested paediatrician (I do a combined clinic with a paediatric endocrinologist every 2 months).

Question 42. A growing problem

Two very short parents – father 4 ft 11 in and mother 4 ft 10 in – have always felt their stature to be a disadvantage. Are there any circumstances in which you might consider giving their child growth hormone? Bearing in mind the recent tragedies with growth hormone is there now any danger in the products used?

I do use growth hormone. It is now safe.

Depending on the size of the child, I would have to consider using growth hormone, if necessary, because the parental sizes here are 2.5 standard deviations from the norm (especially father). The parents could easily have a dyschondroplastic syndrome and growth hormone and other growth promoting factors are now being tried on some of these conditions. Other forms of treatment such as leg-lengthening surgery have shown success, and I would certainly have the whole family assessed.

Growth hormone is now synthetic and no longer contains the viral threat posed by cadaver pituitary.

Question 43. How long does a premature infant take to catch up?

A doctor is carrying out developmental checks at 6 weeks and 18 months. He sees a number of children who have been premature, some markedly so. Is there a rule of thumb on how this might affect their various milestones? How long does the premature infant take to catch up?

The most important calculation is brainday age.

The very preterm infant has two ages, a birthday age and a brainday age. Can the brain's neurodevelopmental processes really be speeded up by being born early? Does bombardment of the visual, auditory and other sensory (e.g. introducing gravity, pain) pathways hinder or enhance development? Much has been written but I believe the practising clinician is best able to judge normality (and deviation from it) by comparing like with like.

I would do a developmental check on the infant born at 26 weeks gestation i.e. 14 weeks premature, at 20 weeks (brainday age 6 weeks), 44 weeks (brainday age 30 weeks) and 66 weeks (brainday age 52 weeks).

The major milestones scored by primary care doctors and nurses are in fact motor ones and using the above 'addition' dates will mean fewer infants are deemed abnormal on a delay basis.

Of course the very early baby is the one at greatest risk of developmental delay and abnormality, so beware. After 1 year normal developmental variations are even wider, e.g. speech etc., so that the pre-term factor plays less part in fogging issues.

Some functions are well documented as being speeded up by early birth, e.g. social smiling.

I am always happy to see positive neurodevelopmental achievements ahead of time, but the real point is when should you worry if they have not appeared. Allowing the times, as above, will avoid you making mistakes that may unnecessarily trouble an already vulnerable family (as anyone who has endured neonatal intensive or special care must be).

Except in the case of extreme prematurity, or in those cases where the prematurity has been associated with chronic on-going illness, I would expect most premature infants to be generally indistinguishable from their peers at the end of the first year, though the trained paediatrician should notice differences for some time after.

Question 44.   The first bed, pillow and walk upstairs

At what age and at what stage in development should a child be moved from cot to bed? Be given a pillow? Be allowed to go up and down stairs unattended?

Parent's instincts are usually the best guide to these decisions.

Truby King, Spock, Brazelton, Jolly – we always seem to revert to some charismatic figure to tell parents what to do. I prefer to point out indicators for parents to draw their own conclusions:

* Would you keep your child in a cot if he climbs enough to threaten he can go over the top?

Fortunately, some wise manufacturers have taken the legs off cots and you can even have removable bars in these floor-standing versions. Then the toddler works out how to take them out before the parent.

* When the child is big enough to cope with a bed he surely is big enough to cope with a pillow. Of course you could put a 'safe' pillow in the cot as soon as the infant is able to roll over, but he is as likely to put it on his head as under it. Is there any point in using one?
* Children should be taught and encouraged to acquire skills as soon as possible. This is a parental joy and responsibility and

great care should be taken to ensure the child is protected until seen to be clearly competent. I would ask the parent what had already been achieved and would be on the look-out for 'reckless drivers', but in the main parents are good judges of their child's competence. The age of 'consent' varies enormously.

Question 45. When is puberty precocious?

A girl of 9½ years is brought to the surgery by her mother. The mother is very concerned that the girl has started breast development and has just had a period. Would this be an abnormally young age to start puberty? If not, when would be? What should be done in the way of investigation if there was precocious puberty? Are there any ethnic differences?

This would be an abnormally young age to start the menarche and I would have grave concern about the possibility of stunted growth.

It is very difficult to define the parameters of normal puberty. The sequences are very variable, and the onset and duration of each element of puberty shows a wide range. Figure 6 illustrates relevant events as described in a Caucasian cohort some 20 years ago. It is seen that:

- Breast development starting at 9½ years appears in less than 5% of girls, the usual time of onset being around 11 years.
- Pubic hair stages very closely match breast development changes.
- Fewer than 3% started their periods before 11 years: the average onset of menarche was 13 years.
- The maximum growth rate occurs at 12 years of age for most, with less than 3% reaching this fast peak before 10 years.

So your young lady poses a number of problems. Decisions on whether physiological or pathological processes are at work require a more complete individual assessment (Figure 6).

Examination would focus on the other secondary sexual characteristics, the thyroid (e.g. hypothyroidism can cause precocious puberty), skin (e.g. pigmentary changes of McCune–Albright syndrome), the CNS including head circumference, fundoscopy and visual fields (e.g. pituitary tumour, severe epilepsy) and abdomen (e.g. hepatic and ovarian tumour). The growth rate of the child with the parental heights must be appropriately charted. Father's height (F) plotted on the growth chart has 13 cm deducted (Fd) (Figure 7).

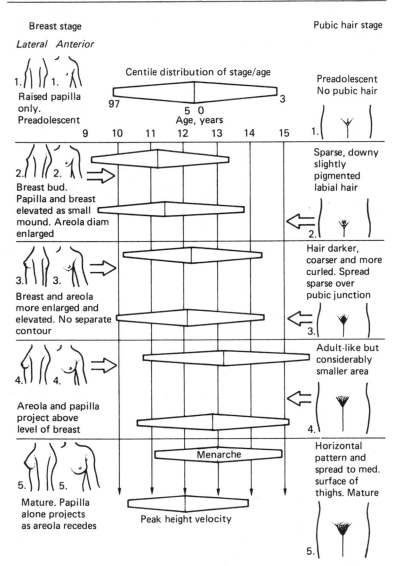

Figure 6 Puberty in girls: As can be seen, more than 97 girls out of every 100 would not have had a period under the age of 11 years

It must be emphasized that there is precocious puberty (patho-logical) and physiological early puberty. The latter is very often family related. Thus a well grown girl having her first period at

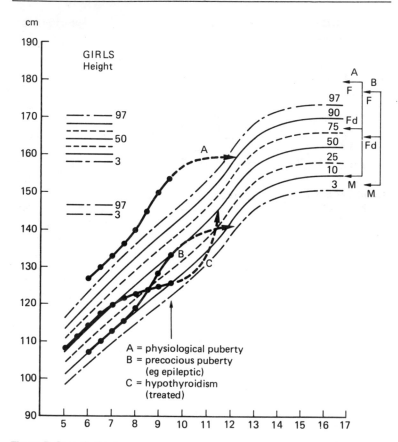

cm

GIRLS
Height

A = physiological puberty
B = precocious puberty
(eg epileptic)
C = hypothyroidism
(treated)

Figure 7 Growth chart

11 years (as did her mother before her) will reach her expected targets, whereas a small child who has a period, unexpectedly, at the same age probably will not.

The investigations the paediatricians would carry out would include visual fields, abdominal ultrasound, X-rays (lateral skull for pituitary fossa, wrist for bone age) and blood tests including electrolytes, thyroid and adrenal hormones and, quite possibly, examination, under general anaesthetic, of genitalia to exclude cervical or vaginal tumour.

There can be ethnic differences in the onset of puberty but these are not, generally, particularly significant.

In this case, unless I could explain the reason for all the signals of early puberty, I would be concerned that she was heading for a severe degree of stunted growth.

Question 46. Extreme prematurity. What is the prognosis?

An extremely premature child is born to a young couple. They seek the advice of their doctor on whether or not the child, if he/she survives, is likely to be severely disabled. Is there a degree of prematurity below which, almost invariably, significant disability occurs – particularly involving the respiratory system – and a degree above which expectation approximates to the full-term infant?

A child of <1000 g (27/28 weeks) has a 12% chance of surviving to be totally normal, a child of >2500 g (35 weeks) has expectations closely approximating to a full term infant.

Birthweight is more objective than gestational age. Modern neonatal intensive care is such a dynamic speciality that each change in practice may influence outcome and it is now difficult to give clear prognoses. Table 4 has been extrapolated from the Scottish Low Birthweight study of all infants born weighing less than 1750 g in 1984 assessed at 4½ years. These results are probably of more significance than the usual descriptions of outcome from a single 'show case' unit.

Survival of premature babies

	<1000 g	1000–1499 g	1500–1749 g
Number of births	204	398	294
% dead by 1 month	62%	18%	7%
% dead by 4 years	70%	21%	10%

Impairment of survivors at 4½ years

	<1000 g	1000–1499 g	1500–1749 g
Unimpaired	42%	54%	58%
Impaired. Not disabled	25%	30%	27%
Moderately disabled	20%	11%	9%
Severely disabled	13%	5%	6%

Thus to put it in its simplest terms, of 100 babies born at a weight of under 1000 g only 30 survived to the age of 4½ years. Of those, 12 were unimpaired, 7 were impaired but not disabled, 6 were moderately disabled and 5 were severely disabled.

Impairment without disability. Neuromotor signs but no functional loss (awkwardness); visual acuity 6/18–6/24; hearing loss ≤ 40 dB; IQ 70–84.

Moderate disability. Cerebral palsy in which the child can sit, stand or walk with aids; vision corrects to 6/36 to 6/60; hearing loss 40–55 dB in best ear without aids; IQ 50–69.

Severe disability. Cerebral palsy in which the child *cannot* sit, stand or walk independently, is blind or with an acuity less than 6/60 in the best eye; or deaf or hearing loss greater than 55 dB; overall IQ less than 50.

From these findings, therefore, you could tell the parents:

- If their baby is 1000 g or less (1000 g being about the average for a 27–28 week gestational aged baby), the babe will have a 30% chance of surviving and if survives, a 40% chance of freedom from neurological abnormality, i.e. a *total of 12% normal outcome*.
- Chronic lung disease (oxygen dependency beyond 28 days) is on the increase as very low birthweight babies survive. Some 70% of infants birthweight <1000 g may develop bronchopulmonary dysplasia (BPD). They may have frequent respiratory problems thereafter, especially in the first 1–2 years, but some have changes in the lung that persist to adulthood.
- After 35 weeks gestation (weight 2500 g) modern expectations would closely approximate to that of the full term infant.

Remember term = 40 ± 2 week, i.e. from end of 37 weeks to beginning of 42 weeks.

Question 47.   Active, well, but no weight gain

A little girl of 2½ years is brought to the doctor. She is very active and appears quite well but her mother is most anxious that she has not put on any weight 'for months'. The doctor reassures the mother that, sometimes, children of this age can, indeed, go for long periods of time without noticeable weight gain. After how long should he begin to get concerned?

Weight gain is not an accurate guide to good health in a toddler. Six months is the kind of period of time before I would begin to look for a cause in an apparently healthy child.

It may help (doctor and parents) to realize the problem of using weight at this stage as an indicator of good health. Reading the standard Tanner and Whitehouse growth chart for girls, aged 0–19 years shows that (Table 4) a small, but perfectly normal 2-year-old gains 1.7 kg (60 ounces) in the forthcoming year, believe it or not, some *5 ounces* (150 g) per month. The variation in daily body weight is considerably influenced by:

- Being erect, or sleeping via an effect on water control.
- Feeding/starvation status.

Table 4. Standard weight (and height) gains

	3rd percentile	50th percentile	97th percentile
Weight, aged 3 years	11.5 kg	14.5 kg	17.7 kg
Weight, aged 2 years	9.8 kg	12.3 kg	15.1 kg
Total weight-gain 2nd to 3rd birthday	1.7 kg (60 oz)	2.2 kg (70 oz)	2.6 kg (92 oz)
Height, aged 3 years	85.5 cm	92.5 cm	100.0 cm
Height, aged 2 years	78.5 cm	84.5 cm	90.5 cm
Total height increase 2nd to 3rd birthday	7.0 cm (2¾")	8.0 cm (3⅛")	9.5 cm (3¾")

- Presence of empty/full bladder or rectum.
- Accuracy and standardization of scales used.

Where growth is rapid, particularly in the first 6 months of life, weight increments are relatively high and the variations indicated represent a small percentage of error. *Beyond the age of 1 year, for reasons illustrated, weight becomes a poor indicator of good health.* Head circumference (with metal or paper tape) can be more accurately followed; length on a stadiometer (see Question 35) can be measured with fewer variations (and the increments are larger); arm circumference on an individual child indicates fat thickness change (used frequently in developing countries); skinfold calipers can be even more accurate but require skill training.

In the well child, as gauged by history and examination, the target size may be influenced by knowledge of parental size. If increments of height, and head circumference follow previous percentile lines but weight remains static then I would show the parents the explanations above and ask to remeasure the child at 3-monthly intervals (same observer).

I would counsel:

- Not to force feed and not to feed between meal-times.
- To encourage self-feeding at meal-times, surrounding the child with people enjoying their food (especially other children) but *not* focusing on feeding others.
- To avoid 'compensating' untaken meals with 'sops' or 'junk food' that the child will happily scoff and beg for between meals. Good eating may be rewarded, not bad habits, i.e. 'if you eat your dinner you can have crisps, if you can't eat your dinner you can't be hungry!'

- To try to reduce fluid intake if the attention-seeking polydipsia typical of this age group seems to be blunting appetite.

I might ask a dietitian colleague to analyse a typical week's diary of intake, type and amount, fluid and solid, kept by a parent. This is particularly helpful in assessing calorie intake as well as adequacy of calcium, iron and vitamins (there are computer programs to make this task easier). I would have a low threshold for checking for anaemia (see Question 50) and eliminating urine infection (but the latter is not such a common cause of failure to thrive as in an infant). With no other clues or indicators, it would take at least two further measurements of weight in the wrong direction (i.e. 6 months) to shatter my confidence.

Question 48.   Bandy and pin-toed

A toddler of 18 months has been walking for some time. He looks well and there is no problem with his nutrition. His mother says that he seems very bandy and pin-toed, 'often tripping over his feet'. Should there be any cause for concern?

A degree of bandiness or knock-knee or pin-toeing is normal and will correct itself.

Being rolled up in a ball for the last 3 months of intrauterine life, even in a 'normal' presentation, flexes and abducts the hips, crosses the tibiae and squashes the feet. The femoral head grows at an angle quite out of keeping with the upright stance. No wonder this gives rise to:

- Anteversion (limiting internal rotation) or retroversion (limiting external rotation) of the femoral head giving 'pin-toeing' and 'duck-waddling', respectively.
- Lateral bowing of the tibiae, giving a bandy or bent look.
- Various degrees of postural (correctable) talipes together with metatarsus varus, the forefoot displacement.

To these may be added a degree of knock-knee, a common finding in the child when first walking, mainly due to lax ligaments around the knee joints accentuating mild fetal compression effects. Nearly all of these are minor and self-correcting and the previous practices of splinting, special moulds in shoes, etc. have been abandoned. It is important to examine all the joints of the legs to ensure these are correctable variations and not fixed or associated with dislocations e.g. of the hip – hopefully an unlikely finding at this age with all the screening that should have occurred in early months.

It is all a matter of degree. A paediatric orthopaedic surgeon, when asked at what stage he surgically intervened in a case of talipes equinovarus, once commented that he really began to get concerned when the upper surface of the shoe became more worn than the sole!

Question 49. Unnecessary circumcision

A little boy of 2½ years is brought by the father who thinks the child needs a circumcision. On examination, the doctor finds that the foreskin does not retract at all and the father confirms that he has tried to retract the foreskin at bathtime with no result. The little boy has no symptoms, is dry and has never had balanitis. Is the operation necessary?

Neither necessary, nor advisable.

The mucosal reflection from the foreskin to glans is very distal in the newborn. It can take many years, in excess of 5 (often 10), for that reflection to develop proximally and allow preputial retraction to occur spontaneously (Figure 8).

It is common advice, in the name of 'genital hygiene', for the parents to be asked to attempt gentle retraction from an early age. Much of that advice comes from health workers. All this will result in is tearing of the fragile mucosal sulcus and may well lead to scarring and phimosis, creating the very cause for circumcision the procedure is supposed to avoid. Retraction should be left to the child himself, at a time he can understand, knowing he will not go beyond what is comfortable.

The case for circumcision on medical grounds has again come under intense scrutiny in the USA. It is possible to pick large holes in the evidence that purports:

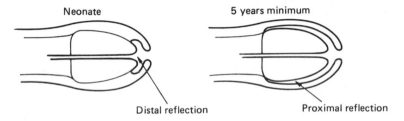

Figure 8 The development of the mucosal reflection

- Reduced phimosis, balanitis and improved genital hygiene.
- Decreased incidence of penile cancer.
- The incidence of cervical cancer might be reduced.
- Decrease in sexually transmitted disease in later years.
- Decreased incidence of urinary tract infection in early months.

The case against circumcision counts:

- The risk of post-operative infected wounds.
- The risks of post-operative bleeding.
- The risks of mistakes especially as surgery is often delegated to relatively inexperienced operators.
- The pain and anguish or
- The risk of general anaesthetic.
- The cost–benefit ratio.

The vitamin K controversy (1992) that may influence current practice for prophylaxis against haemorrhagic disease of the newborn could prove another serious factor against neonatal surgical procedures.

No operation needed for medical reasons is my counsel to the father.

Question 50.   How significant is a low haemoglobin?

At what level of haemoglobin would you start treating a child of (a) 2 years, (b) 5 years, (c) 10 years with oral iron? Is a low haemoglobin in a child so often dietary that further investigations are unnecessary? Is routine haemoglobin estimation in growing children a reasonable health promotion exercise?

It depends very much on the level – and the age.

There are a number of factors that influence the haemoglobin pre-term, at delivery and post-term. The fetus gathers iron with great rapidity in the last trimester and leaving base camp early denies a large part of this supply. At birth 35–75 mg iron are available in the placenta and the amount received by the baby may depend largely on how early, or late, the cord is clamped. After birth the fetal haemoglobin is gradually replaced by adult haemoglobin and the Hb level falls from 18 g to 11 g. This iron is not lost but stored. Rapid growth, particularly in a low weight baby, will rapidly diminish these stores. Breast milk, adequate initially, falls in iron content after 6 months. Cow's milk iron is not absorbed very effectively and unadulterated milk can cause some blood loss from the infant gut.

Table 5. Symptoms and signs of iron deficiency

Basic problem	Clinical situation	
Diminished stores	Preterm delivery	
	Placental transfer loss	
Rapid growth	Early infancy esp. if low birth weight	
Poor intake	Nutritional factors – Quantitative	
	– Qualitative	
	– Complex	
Inefficient absorption	Chronic inflammatory diseases	
	Malabsorption syndromes	
Increased losses	Gastro-intestinal, e.g.	Meckel's
		Polyps
		Cows' milk allergy
		Parasites
		Drugs, e.g. NSAID
	Non-gastro-intestinal, e.g.	Nose bleeds
		Menorrhagia

As a result of these factors the amount of iron available to the baby might be less than required and a microcytic anaemia results.

Although a microcytic anaemia is most commonly caused by iron deficiency in this country, there is an important differential diagnosis:

• Disorders of globin synthesis, e.g. thalassaemia traits.
• Anaemias of chronic disorders, e.g. inflammatory diseases such as juvenile chronic arthritis, Crohn's disease, malignancy.
• Lead poisoning.

Even if iron deficiency emerges as the likely cause of the microcytic anaemia, giving iron therapy might not attack the root of the problem (see Table 5).

Now I can specifically approach the questions.

A haemoglobin of less than 10 g/dl must be considered abnormal at all ages referred to, but will represent a more significant anaemia at 10 years and only just significant at 2 years of age. I would counsel all doctors to request *every* blood count they ask for on children in the following manner:

If the haemoglobin is less than 10 g/dl or the MCV is less than 75(fl) then please also perform haemoglobin electrophoresis, serum iron and total iron binding capacity (or ferritin level for some labs). This can be simply written: 'If Hb <10 or MCV <75 please do serum iron, TIBC and Hb electrophoresis'. Enough blood is then taken at the *first* venesection; but the extra tests are only performed if the Hb/MCV indicate.

A high incidence of thalassaemia traits is found in the Asian community. The common form of β-thalassaemia trait will show a high level of HbA_2, but the common form of α-thalassaemia trait can be difficult to differentiate from iron deficiency. To worsen matters, many Asian children are also iron deficient.

A good history is the best guide to the need for other investigations: ethnic background for other haemoglobinopathies, foreign residence or travel for stool parasites, atopic features (e.g. eczema) for milk allergy tests; pica for lead levels; gastrointestinal symptoms for radiological studies or jejunal biopsy.

I would never care to give iron therapy, in this country, without having scientific justification. It may be necessary to initiate a trial of iron therapy for some weeks to clarify uncertain parameters especially suggestive of α-thalassaemia and iron deficiency combined.

I believe extensive nutritional advice throughout pregnancy and early infancy is a better approach to 'iron health promotion' than traumatizing three-quarters of the childhood population unnecessarily. However, I would have a very low threshold for blood letting in a child from a high risk population, e.g. poor dietary and social milieu, or from the Asian community. Severe iron deficiency in infants must not be missed as the long-term developmental outcome has been repeatedly shown to be markedly adverse.

Table 6. Normal (mean) values

Age (yr)	Weight (kg)	Hb (g/dl) ±2SD	MCV (fl)	HbF (%)	HbA₂ (%)	Serum iron μmol/l	TIBC μmol/l	Transferrin Saturation (%)
2	12–13	12±1.5	81±6	0.25–1.3	1.4–3.3	16	44	34
5	18.5	12.5±1.0	85±9	0.25–1.3	1.4–3.3	15	56	25
10	30	13.5±2.0	86±9	0.25–1.3	1.4–3.3	14	62	24

One final comment on iron therapy – the dose for therapy is 3–5 mg/kg of elemental iron per day. It is wise to stick to one preparation and become familiar with its content of elemental iron avoiding risks of under/over dosage. I use Sytron [55 mg of elemental iron (ferrous) in 10 ml of liquid]. The total dose to be given is divided into 3 aliquots in the day, before food. There is often a marked effect on stool colour and consistency and it is important to verify compliance. Replacing iron stores completely takes months rather than weeks (until MCV returns to >75).

Nervous and neurological

Question 51. Afebrile fits – always epilepsy?

A child of 2 years has a grand mal convulsion. She is apyrexial. There is no family history of epilepsy. What possible diagnoses should be considered and what action should be taken?

There are numerous possibilities but epilepsy is by far the most likely cause.

The overwhelming probability is epilepsy regardless of family history. At this age secondary epilepsy is high on the agenda and a thorough review of pre-, peri- and post-natal events is essential. Precise details from the witness to the event may give vital clues that might distinguish commoner (or rarer) possibilities such as:

- Breath-holding spell.
- Hypoglycaemia (always measure the blood sugar of any unconscious child as soon as possible).
- Accidental drug ingestion.
- Unexpected drug side effect.
- Head injury (accidental or otherwise).

The examination must be meticulous because:

- Infection does not always produce constant pyrexia – look for the petechiae of meningococcus.
- Post-infectious neurological complications are often afebrile, e.g. chicken pox encephalomyelitis – look for lesions.
- Tell-tale signs of abuse are not yet all confined to history books.
- Papilloedema may point the way to the not unusual occurrence of a brain tumour at this age.
- The shagreen patch or depigmentation of tuberose sclerosis may still escape recognition until a more dramatic feature of that disease appears.

A fit in a 2-year-old must be referred and I would wish to see such a child immediately. Of course, if the fit continues for more than 5 minutes, you must take appropriate action – rectal diazepam 5 mg – and arrange for accompanied admission, while the child is kept in the recovery position.

Question 52.   Bed-wetting. Does anything help?

The parents of a 5-year-old child bring him to the doctor concerned that he still wets the bed. It transpires that the mother wet the bed until she was 6 years old and the father until he was 10. Does this make the immediate prognosis hopeless? What measures would you try? Are there any circumstances in which you would use antidiuretic hormone?

It is not hopeless. Various methods can be tried. ADH is useful for short periods.

I would not consider it hopeless just because it takes a while longer to achieve dryness. If everyone, particularly the child, was keen to beat nature's intention then I would try to move things on. Assuming a careful examination and urine check has been done, I would try a star chart and parental lifting of the child before they retired to sleep, to encourage 'mutual' involvement. I would not be averse to using ADH for a few days to 'inspire' confidence but the relapse rate is high. I would try an enuretic alarm fairly soon but ensure no-one is going to be unreasonable in their expectations, demands or disappointments. Motivated families have a high success rate with a buzzer, used properly, with equipment immediately replaced if faulty, and with an enthusiastic 'therapist'.

Sometimes the child is reassured, less guilty, and even more determined to succeed if he finds that his mother and father had the same problem when they were young. Very often this information has never been volunteered by the parents until asked straight out at the time of consultation – not infrequently much to the child's delight!

Although of little use in the long term treatment of bed-wetting, antidiuretic hormone (ADH) can be particularly useful if the child is going on holiday or staying in a strange bed. One puff up each nostril of a product such as Desmospray (vasopressin) an hour before going to bed will probably ensure a dry night. However, do not use for too many nights at a time.

Question 53.   Working class – 'slow': middle class – 'dyslexic'

The 'dyslexic' child almost always seems to have middle-class parents and almost never lives in a multi-storey block of council flats. A GP is faced by the under-achieving son of high-achieving parents and is asked to refer him for correction of 'his condition'.

To whom? What proportion of such cases are children who are, by the law of averages, not as bright as their parents who have no particular discernible – or treatable – pathway difficulties? How might you recognize the genuine article?

Learning difficulties have no social frontier. If there is genuine concern, at whatever level, refer for multidisciplinary assessment.

Most people have difficulty in some aspect of learning. A difficulty focused on one skill may be seen as specific, especially if set in a background of others more accomplished, thus heightening the degree of handicap that ensues.

It is against this background that the specific reading disorder known as dyslexia has to be viewed and is likely to have cultural and socio-economic distortions. Such disabilities can occur without respect for the degree of intelligence. It is quite as disabling for a person with an IQ of 100 to have a reading and spelling ability 30 points below this level as it is for one with an IQ of 130, and its discovery and management, irrespective of social circumstances, is just as important.

Specific learning disorders have to be unravelled from the plethora of causative or contributing factors. Input, cognition and output are complex functions. Vision and visual discrimination (spatial knowledge), hearing and auditory discrimination (listening), memory, imagery, attention, intelligence, physical factors (neuro-motor skills, cerebral dominance factors), behaviour and emotion and social experiences indicate some of the elements that may be pertinent.

Thus a multidisciplinary assessment by professionals who have an interest in such problems and who hopefully pool and discuss their knowledge, and differences, is the favoured approach.

Start with a paediatrician, now often the member of a co-ordinated group of paediatricians, with special interest in educational paediatrics where a careful history, examination and initial investigations are undertaken prior to assessment by speech therapist, occupational and physiotherapist, educational psychologist and teacher. Special senses (vision and hearing) must be checked. The number of people involved and the order of their involvement can best be co-ordinated by teamwork planning.

Many attempts have been made to group types of learning disorders into reading, spelling and mathematical areas with various subgroups. Numbers have been placed on these divisions so decided. I prefer not to think in percentages but to take each concern seriously and use teamwork to expand the details and decide the options, or need, for management.

Most children that end up seeing me tend to be, for one reason or another, the genuine article. I am always alerted by a history of cross-dominance or clumsiness – although these factors now seem less important – but most particularly by a child who appears to operate much more poorly in one area than the rest of his or her profile would suggest.

Question 54.   Temporal lobe or temper?

A boy of 12 is well behaved most of the time but sometimes has bouts of violent, unreasonable behaviour. Some of these bouts are when he cannot get his own way but sometimes there is no explanation. The father is sure the boy is playing up. The mother points out that a distant cousin has temporal lobe epilepsy (TLE). Could one situation mimic the other? Would an EEG give a definitive answer? What clues might point one way or the other – or is it possible that there might be a totally unexpected explanation like solvent abuse?

The situation might be complex but a sleep EEG could be very helpful.

Who would care to define unreasonable behaviour in the adolescent? Parental concern, rarely unanimously agreed, must be responded to, but will the young person agree to participate? Psychomotor epilepsy accounts for about one quarter of all seizures, but there is usually a clear aetiological pointer in two-thirds of cases of TLE (previous brain-damaging illness or chronic neurological disease).

Inheritance only seems to play some part through a predisposition to febrile convulsions in first degree relatives. An early history of status epilepticus from a febrile illness would certainly be relevant.

Psychomotor seizures are usually of short duration, often without precipitating factors, and start and finish suddenly. Although emotional disturbance may provoke seizures, a careful history should point out the stereotyping of the events very different from the pattern of a personality disturbance. Associated behavioural disturbances can occur alongside TLE, particularly hyperkinesis and outbursts of catastrophic rage.

Similar behaviour at school or outside home life might weigh in favour of TLE if all other information fails to convince. Medical explanations for bad behaviour are always favoured by society. How rare it is that drug abuse, family dysharmony and an atrocious school life are disclosed or put 'up front'.

Should doubts exist, a sleep EEG is the most likely to yield helpful information as a one-off test. Between attacks, recordings in children are more likely to show abnormalities than in adults. EEG findings are not specific for epilepsy but are vastly more common in those who have had seizures than those who have not.

Question 55.   No sleep for the parents

The parents of a 3-year-old child comes to the doctor in a state of desperation as their son wakes up at midnight every night and insists on coming into their bed to play for 2 or 3 hours before going back to sleep again. If the child is left in his own room he screams for very long periods and everyone ends up exhausted. What would you advise?

Persuasion or sedation.

There are two courses of action, to induce sleep with drugs or seduce sleep by behavioural modification. I believe in ensuring parental survival and the exhausted family are unlikely to find the concentration and patience it needs to implement a behavioural programme. I thus offer, but am delighted to have refused, trimeprazine 4 mg – yes, 4 mg per kg, rounded down to the lower volume of Vallergan Forte (30 mg in 5 ml) given 45 minutes before settling the child down. The dose may need titrating back but usually the family do not give the full dosage anyway. The child may be drowsy the next morning but at least the family know they have a rescue device. Chloral hydrate elixir, 30–45 mg/kg at night, is an alternative, more unpleasant to taste but with less hangover. In the first event I would give these kind of doses for a week then reduce but, sometimes, high doses have to be maintained for weeks.

At the same time, I introduce the principles behind behavioural modification and search through the attitudes and rituals of the family, discovering the obvious distractions such as father arriving home at midnight and wanting a quick peep, or playing with his long lost child. You need to know if there is only one room, when separation is impossible, or if the baby is the only way sex can be avoided by one partner or the other!

The parents must debate the possibilities and pace of change, ensuring clear distinction between expectations of the child in the day and at night (cueing), gradually employing a separation by · sitting with the child and slowly decreasing contact and with positive reinforcement (reward), e.g. stars or 'in vogue' stickers. 'My child won't sleep' (Penguin 1986) by Jo Douglas and Naomi Richman is helpful reading for parents. A short inservice training with a skilled clinical psychologist is good preparation for doctors.

My aim, therefore, is to revitalize exhausted parents. A week or two of good sleep leads to a gain in control and confidence before attempting the patience, harmony and consistency on which behavioural modification depends. The trimeprazine can slowly be reduced in volume – if necessary by as little as 0.5 ml every 2 or 3 nights – until a minimum threshold is found. Alternatively, the parents might wish to miss out a night's treatment. All that most ask is having an occasional rescue device which, more often than not, is not used.

Question 56. Head banger

A little boy of 2½ years terrifies his parents by banging his head against the wall every time he seeks to attract their attention. Reassured by their GP, they tolerate the situation until the child sustains a large bump on the forehead following a demonstration against a recently tiled bathroom wall. Should they be advised to continue to ignore these tantrums? Do children ever sustain significant head injury or brain damage by this kind of head banging?

Continue to reassure. He is very unlikely to come to any serious harm.

It is probably a way of letting off steam or ritualistically resolving tension and is said to occur in 1 in 20 children of this age. I have never seen a significant injury and it is to be remembered that children hit their heads much harder without harm in other escapades.

Assuming no other serious disease is present that might make head banging a danger – a bleeding diathesis, brittle bones, etc. – I too, would be reassuring.

In this case the child probably made an error of judgement and will not repeat this particular exercise again. Children usually choose surfaces that resound fiercely and give a spectacular result rather than stony ones that don't make much noise and hurt!

Question 57. Spare the rod, it spoils the child

To smack or not to smack? Are there any indications? Are there any particular contraindications? Should the blow, if at all, be delivered in the heat of the moment or retrospectively? On what portion of the anatomy? In what circumstances would you contact

a social worker if you found finger shaped bruises on the back of a child's calves?

Avoid smacking if possible. Bruising from smacking would be a worrying sign of excessive force.

I would rather help the parents adopt other methods of controlling their children, but smacking is rife in our society. A parent who has the overall view of events may choose to underline disapproval of dangerous or serious misdemeanours at the time by a smack on the bottom (over clothes) or legs. A child in a loving relationship, and with a parent who explains the reason for the reprimand, and who quickly forgives the child, is unlikely to be harmed.

Impetuous, uncontrolled lashing out, wrenching of limbs, pulling and shaking may be extremely dangerous especially to infants and young children. Such actions can lead to whiplash and contra-coup injuries to the brain apart from well recognized torsion injuries around the shoulders and knees. It is important to have a sensitive and empathetic understanding of all the circumstances, but if doubts exist you must make time to talk it through with the family or discuss it with someone with the time and skill to do it for you (preferably a social worker with special skills in child abuse work).

I must admit I would worry if the hitting was hard enough to impose bruising, especially if it happened more than once and the parents were unwilling to explain how and why.

Question 58. Mayhem in the surgery

A mother returns to the surgery after a visit to the paediatrician. As usual, her 3-year-old is quite unmanageable and it is only with great difficulty that the doctor can desist from swatting him behind the ear with a copy of MIMS. The mother cannot understand why the paediatrician has given her an amphetamine for her demoniacally active child. 'Surely it's a stimulant, isn't it, Doctor? He'll just never stop at all'. Are her worries justified?

Probably.

I am more worried about the doctor. I don't think hyperkinetic syndrome can be so easily distinguished in the scenario of mild chaos that presents in most doctor's waiting rooms and surgeries – and out-patients! Studies in the UK show a 30-fold, or more, lower incidence of hyperkinetic syndrome than in the USA, throwing some doubt on the reliability of such a diagnosis.

Ask for a few Maudsley profiles on the subject. Like dyslexia, it is seen to be a multifactorial problem and requires careful dissection before resorting to any therapy – especially one as potent as amphetamine.

I agree with the mother on this. Amphetamine does work, by a paradoxical effect to that which the mother fears, in a few well chosen cases, but they have to be very well chosen.

Question 59. 'He needs his sleep, doesn't he, Doctor?'

The mother of a 5-year-old boy is distressed that her son rarely goes to sleep before midnight, preferring to play and look at books. He wakes at 6.30 every morning apparently well and refreshed. Is there a particular amount of sleep a child 'needs' at any given age or do children vary enormously taking the amount of sleep they individually require?

Nobody has ever committed themself on this. Probably wisely!

My suggestion would be for the parents to tell this young man, 'We are quite happy that you can't sleep, but you must read quietly for we do need *our* sleep'.

No late meal or TV, a strenuous bit of exercise, a warm bath or shower and restful reading are all useful rituals to encourage good diurnal rhythms, which, although dependent on CNS maturation, are also influenced by how much and what sort of stimulation is fed in.

I have looked for norms at this age, but whoever has done the work has not put it in the best read books or journals.

Question 60. Anterior fontanelle – window on intracranial pressure

A very sharp-eyed mother brings her 9-month-old baby to the surgery with a bulging fontanelle, nothing else. The child seems fairly well except there is a history of a little irritability the day before. The child is sent to the paediatric department and much to everybody's surprise turns out to have a viral meningitis. Is the fontanelle frequently overlooked?

No examination of a child under 2 years should exclude the anterior fontanelle.

Alliteratively 'you may be fooled by a full fontanelle but folly if you forget to feel it in the first place'. No clinician to children is a safe one unless he/she routinely measures and checks by chart the head circumference (using paper or steel tape rather than 'stretchy' linen) and feels the anterior fontanelle in all under 2s (usually closed at 18 months). It is even better if the doctor checks the surface of the skull and sutures. A number of pathologies might show up, from early hydrocephalus to unanticipated injury.

The anterior fontanelle is nature's window on raised intracranial pressure and a bulging fontanelle, excepting where the child is 'valsalva-ing' – crying, straining, etc. – should be looked into for causes such as:

- Infections – meningitis, encephalitis, abscess – bacterial infections may be modified by existing antibiotic therapy.
- Subdural collections – perinatal, accidental and non-accidental injury (especially from shaking), bleeding diseases.
- Hypernatraemic dehydration. The fontanelle bulges! Difficult to diagnose.
- Cerebral oedema – hydrocephalus, intracranial haemorrhages, poisons, e.g. lead and carbon monoxide, fluid overload (perhaps from ADH – iatrogenic or from a tumour), hypoxaemia, trauma.
- Benign intracranial hypertension from chronic middle ear disease, drugs, steroid withdrawal, after some head injury.
- Venous sinus thrombosis, especially hyperviscosity in neonatal period.

Remember, a normal fontanelle in a child expected to have a sunken one, e.g. a child who is dehydrated from vomiting, may represent raised intracranial pressure.

Patting the baby's head is more than a friendly gesture.

Question 61. When is a headache significant?

A little girl of 6 years comes to the surgery for the third time in 3 weeks with a headache. There is nothing in her history, neither physical nor psychological, nor in the family history to explain this. Nothing abnormal is found on examination. Should the doctor now refer? If so how urgently?

If there is a significant cause there will usually be at least one other clue, but if in doubt 'soon' referral would be justified.

Another way of looking at this difficult problem is to review the features found in a large group of children with headache due to brain tumour:

- Abnormal neurological signs appear in most cases *within 8 weeks* of the onset of their first symptom (usually headache). The signs to be looking for are:
    (i) Visual acuity loss.
    (ii) Visual field loss.
    (iii) Papilloedema.
    (iv) Lateral rectus palsy.
    (v) Short stature/poor growth rate.
    (vi) Large head (>90th percentile or head considerably greater than length percentile).
    (vii) Cranial bruit.
    (viii) Head tilt.
    (ix) Ataxia.
    (x) Polydipsia (suggesting diabetis insipidus).
    (xi) Bedwetting (secondary)

    apart from the more conventional neurological assessment.

- Behaviour changes are often present early (and almost always identified with other signs mentioned above) *within 4 months* of onset:
    (i) Worsening concentration
    (ii) Slower intellectual progress compared to previous assessments.
    (iii) Changed learning pattern.
    (iv) Apathy ⎫
    (v) Depression ⎬ personality changes
    (vi) Mood swings ⎭

- Features of the headache itself:
    (i) Especially appearing in the under 5s.
    (ii) Recent onset, prolonged pain.
    (iii) Change in nature, frequency and severity.
    (iv) Occurring in the night, awakening child from sleep, or appearing early morning.
    (v) Provoked by coughing or sneezing, or exercise, or lying down.
    (vi) Accompanied by nausea/vomiting/sudden drowsiness/mood change.
    (vii) Not relieved by analgesics.

Using this database, I would recommend your patient has two unusual features; the three attacks in 3 weeks without obvious explanation and the persistence of the pain.
I would therefore

- Take a fuller history and a longer look using the information supplied and rethink; or

- Ask a paediatrician (or paediatric neurologist if you are privileged locally) to do this for you within 2 weeks; or
- Take another look 1–2 weeks later yourself, but finding more details from the school, and telling the parents you want to know if there are any adverse changes.

Accident and emergency

Question 62.   Fall from a window

A mother phones the surgery. Her 5-year-old daughter has fallen from an upstairs window and is unconscious on the patio. What immediate advice would you give her as she awaits the doctor and/or ambulance?

Above all, not to leave the child.

Try to explain the 'recovery' position, achieved with the minimum amount of disturbance especially holding the head with gentle traction from the body as she turns the child onto her side, preferably with assistance. She should not try to carry the child inside, but can cover her child with a coat/blanket provided she does not have to leave the child alone to obtain these.

Without an adequate airway all may be lost regardless of other risks due to other injuries. Spinal injuries in children seem uncommon relative to height of fall. Mouth to mouth should be attempted, after wiping the airway clear, quickly, if there is no spontaneous breathing.

Best of all, on the principles of 'be prepared', persuade all young mothers to learn some first aid so that in certain circumstances they would know what to do straight away – burns, asphyxia, etc. The recovery position can be learned as a game with their own toddler in case it is ever needed.

Question 63.   Swallowing a Goodyear

A doctor is telephoned because a child of 3 years has swallowed a plastic wheel from a toy car. After a short period of dysphagia the child feels perfectly well. 'If it goes down, it will go through'. True or false?

Generally true.

I think a small round wheel that causes no choking or stridor will enter the stomach and if it reaches there 'it is past its worst'. It is important to know precisely what went down by looking at a facsimile if possible, as people's concept of small and large cannot be taken at face value, especially with things like battery sizes (remember with batteries that their contents can pose other problems).

If in doubt, an X-ray will demonstrate the resting place of most radio-opaque objects. Not all objects reaching the stomach are safe, and open pointed objects, e.g. open safety pins, may need endoscopic removal. To avoid unnecessary X-rays, if the object is known to be metal, some units are using metal detectors in these circumstances.

Question 64. Protocol for poisons

What are the most dangerous of the common household liquids that might be drunk by children? Are there any circumstances in which a child should be induced to vomit straight away? If so, how? Are there any plants or trees you would actively discourage in the garden where young children might play? Which adult medications are those most commonly taken accidentally by small children, leading to hospital admission?

A toddler has no appreciation of toxicology. Always have ipecacuanha to hand. Always hospitalize or consult.

- Bleaching agents (sodium hypochlorite solutions), e.g. disinfectants, nappy sterilizers, some denture cleaners are alkaline chemicals, as are many surface cleaning agents containing ammonia. They are thus corrosive, the severity of injury depending on both concentration of solution and the duration of contact. DON'T INDUCE VOMITING.
- Hydrocarbons, e.g. white spirit, window cleaners, turpentine substitute, paraffin and petrol destroy pulmonary surfactant if aspirated, and if absorbed in quantity can produce serious CNS toxicity. Essential oils behave similarly, e.g. camphorated oils, oil of turpentine found in rubs and creams. DON'T INDUCE VOMITING.
- Alcohols can be found in surgical spirit, perfumes, aftershaves, eau-de-Cologne as well as in the VAT 69 bottle – in childhood they produce hypoglycaemia and metabolic acidosis as well as the better known CNS effects. Methanol in model aircraft fuels, screenwashes and some thinners can produce an intense metabolic acidosis. INDUCED VOMITING HELPS.
- Ethylene glycol in antifreezes intoxicates first and leads to acute renal failure later. INDUCED VOMITING HELPS.
- Paraquat weedkiller is hopefully disappearing from old garden sheds. Its toxicity exceeds its corrosive dangers and immediate emesis is necessary. Modern preparations (for the farm) now include an emetic. INDUCED VOMITING HELPS.

In general, corrosives, hydrocarbons and essential oils are too hazardous to the lungs to recommend immediate induction of vomiting.

Spirits and wines often induce emesis themselves if drunk by children but early vomiting is important therapy here. *P*-Dichlorbenzene is used in many toilet cleaning agents, but is not corrosive like bleach. Ingestion should be treated by emesis.

N.B. I note *less* rather than more information on current household liquid containers. It is vital to have your local Poisons Unit telephone number always available and to use it, as details are important.

I believe that every doctor's surgery (and emergency bag) should contain syrup of ipecacuanha. A dose of 15 ml should be given as soon as possible followed by 200 ml of water, and the child jogged up and down, e.g. on a rocking horse or lap. If he/she has not vomited within 15 minutes of the dose, the dose (and ritual) is repeated. Although a rare event, failure to produce vomiting 15 minutes after a second attempt makes gastric lavage essential.

Attractive berries, poisonous and non-poisonous, could arguably be excluded from gardens. Is it fair or logical to encourage scrumptious raspberries while attempting to explain holly berries are dangerous? Only a future Capability Brown is likely to be smart enough at the right age to appreciate the differences. I would not grow deadly or woody nightshade, Christmas cherry, snowberry by choice, but laburnum, yew, holly, foxglove are everywhere as is woody nightshade, common in many hedgerows, with its succulent red berries beckoning any toddler who can reach. I think it is better to ensure the child is properly minded or the gardener's efforts should be directed to constructing a contained area of grass for the vulnerable young to learn to play rugby on. Young children often sample a bit of agriculture, mostly without serious problem, and if emesis is used rapidly should they have obtained a possible poisonous plant, mushroom or berry they are unlikely to be harmed and will have (sadly) had aversion therapy. The vomitus can be used for identification purposes to direct further action if necessary. Always collect any suspicious item of ingested substance – chemical or plant – for careful identification and review once the initial panic is over.

All of the above applies to handling possible or actual ingestion of adult medicines. Prevention is better than cure. All healthcare workers, particularly health visitors and GPs *should ask to see* where medicines and potential toxins are kept in the home where young children might live or visit. It should be in a place difficult for adults to reach, or easily lockable for disabled persons, and blister packs to delay access time should be encouraged.

The current major hospital 'ingestion' Top of the Pops list is:

- CNS drugs – antidepressants (increasing), anxiolytics (lessening).
- Analgesics – salicylates and other non-steroidal anti-inflammatory drugs (half the world).
- Cardiovascular – antiarrhythmics, antihypertensives in all their rich varieties (in grandma's handbag).
- Iron preparations (everywhere in pregnant mothers' homes apart from the first pregnancy!).

I guess that the easiest way to check future incidence will be for paediatricians to have copies of PACT prescribing lists from the contracted fund holding GPs!

Question 65. The tight toddler

A doctor is called at Christmas time to see a little boy of 5 years who has drunk an unknown quantity of sweet sherry and when seen is quite intoxicated, i.e. staggering and slurring his speech (the child, not the doctor). Should he be hospitalized? Would your answer be different if the child had drunk an unknown quantity of (a) a table wine? (b) a sweet liqueur?

If he is intoxicated, admit, whatever his tipple!

Yes, admit such children. Alcohol in all its guises is much more dangerous at this age. There is a strong possibility of hypoglycaemia as a part of acute intoxication, apart from severe CNS depression with its attendant worries of respiratory depression and possible aspiration of vomitus. It is our practice to give IV dextrose to intoxicated children. They usually have 'drug induced' emesis before or by the time they reach us.

Question 66. The inexperienced carer

An unmarried woman of 35 is looking after her sister's 3-year-old child whilst the child's mother is in hospital. She has never looked after a toddler before and is extremely anxious that no harm should befall him. What are the commonest accidents that happen to children of toddler age and how might they best be avoided?

She will probably be a lot more careful than the parents!

Her anxieties should be higher if given a nephew to guard rather than a niece. She should have her wits about her most when she ventures outside the house where 38% of accidental deaths occur in road traffic accidents (RTAs) in those under 4 years of age. Next comes death by drowning, submersion or suffocation (20%); by burning in fire and flames (17%) and in falls (7%). Obviously these are also major causes of serious accidents short of fatality. Add to this list, poisoning and we can reduce this poor aunt to hysterics.

But life is not like that. Most adults have marvellous protective instincts for the young and aunties everywhere should play a role in helping their family with lots of joy and enthusiasm, and little fear.

Two further comments should be made, however. She will not possess the four hands that all mothers develop whilst going around the supermarket – the hand to push the trolley, the hand to hold the child, the hand to take things off the shelf and the hand to put things back that the toddler has taken off. If the mother has two or more small children she will develop six hands. Auntie can make up for this by using reins on the child. Indeed, for any carer of small children these out-of-fashion appliances are invaluable to stop them dashing out into the road which, as mentioned, is the greatest danger of all.

If the child is staying with Auntie, it is easy for something as deadly dangerous as a tiny, apparently harmless, fish pond to be overlooked. Children have drowned in an inch or two of water. The whole geography of the child's temporary home must be looked at with the eye of someone 36 inches tall!

Question 67.   Accident prone or abused?

For the third time in 5 months a child is brought to see the doctor with a significant injury. On this occasion it is a large bump on the head from 'falling off a chair'. The previous events were a greenstick fracture of the radius (another fall) and an injury to the fingers (caught in a door). The doctor is loath to make a diagnosis of non-accidental injury as the parents seem loving and caring. Are some children more accident prone than others? If so, how do you tell them apart from children who are subject to non-accidental injury?

Some children are more accident prone than others and sometimes there is lack of care rather than deliberate abuse.

Accident proneness is a disease entity itself and is probably one area of impaired parental care-taking. For this reason it is sometimes known as 'the vulnerable child syndrome'. It can happen when the parental anxieties and energies are being displaced or diverted from appropriate child-rearing by situations such as financial worry, marital breakdown and conditions like depression where the mother may be insufficiently motivated to look after the child properly. In a history like the one above, the age of the child is most important. The most serious cases are those that involve children less than one year old.

A real indicator of actual abuse, that should arouse all warning signals, is a delay in bringing the injured child to the doctor coupled with a description of events that does not tally with the injuries and which includes frequent inconsistencies. This is particularly significant in families known to lack social lifelines, perhaps victims of abuse themselves or known to be under severe stress.

Helping stressed or abusing parents requires knowledge of the dynamics involved. An empathy and desire to help, not condemnation, is more likely to reveal the true dilemma. Any professional dealing with children should have taken part in a multi-disciplinary child abuse course (usually a 2-day affair) when most aspects of non-accidental injury and how each group of professionals can play their part will have been thoroughly explored.

Abdominal problems

Question 68.   The constipated infant

A mother comes to the surgery with her 4-month-old infant. The
child seems much distressed by the passing of large, hard stools.
The mother has tried changing the feeds, giving extra drinks,
giving fruit juices, giving brown sugar and water. She has also
tried glycerine suppositories. All to no avail. How should she
proceed?

Lactulose, patience and relearning.

Many inexperienced parents are concerned at the sight of their
infant's physiological behaviour in raising intra-abdominal
pressure to expel stool. It is difficult to quantify size, consistency
and regularity and all these probably have a biological (Gaussian)
range. At 4 months the introduction of mixed feeding is a
common trigger for changing stool consistency and may be quite
dramatic for the entirely breast-fed infant. If stools are expelled
regularly a few hearty grunts should be accepted and fears
allayed.

However, crying/screaming/bleeding at stool needs action. I will
assume the history does not go back to the neonatal period, for
that raises other uncommon but important issues, e.g. anal
stenoses, malposition or low-segment Hirschsprung's. Most
problems are of short history, following an illness or dietary
change, and often a painful experience such as a fissure perpetu-
ates distress. This may be, in part, a 'conditioned' response rather
than repeated physical pain. Relief must be obtained by a long
spell (weeks/months) of stool softening and I would use Lactulose
(2.5 ml b.d. initially, but increasing if necessary) and continue
increased fluids. It is important to allow enough time for 'relearning' – the rectum contracting down from its acquired distension
and the corticothalamic pathways from their 'negative' feedback.
Pushing things back up the rectum was not nature's intention!

Question 69.   The infant with diarrhoea: should
breast-feeding continue?

A baby of 8 weeks has quite severe diarrhoea. Two other children
in the family have the same complaint. The baby is breast fed and
is extremely reluctant to take feed from any other source, thereby

making it very difficult to use one of the available rehydrating clear fluid preparations. Should the mother just be advised to continue breast-feeding and hope for the best?

If at all possible, try to get the infant on to rehydrating solution for 24 hours, if not, try and give some in addition to the breast milk.

This is a situation to be watched very carefully. Before answering I would like to say that an 8-week baby can be very easily compromised with dehydration and electrolyte disturbance and I would advise that if the child appeared, in any way unwell, 'floppy', pyrexial, vomiting, or with doubtful urinary output, then a paediatric assessment should be sought.

A few preliminary thoughts can be explored. 'Breast-fed infants shouldn't develop gastro-enteritis' – isn't that one of our major propaganda points to enrol nursing mothers? Just check that the mother has not taken the latest herbal remedy to purge herself (wittingly or not) – and the baby. Rarely, a very well baby with a weight gain crossing percentiles upwardly compared to length and head circumference, may just be 'over-feeding' and display diarrhoea. The commonest occurrence will be the commonest agent to cause gastro-enteritis in childhood in the UK, i.e. the rotavirus – often clinically identified by an initial upper respiratory symptomatology including otitis, cough, with very high fever and prolonged profuse diarrhoea (sometimes for 7–10 days whatever dietary manipulations one makes).

It is certainly scientifically studied and has been counselled that breast feeding can be continued under such conditions with excellent outcome. In fact, in the developing nations where concomitant malnutrition abounds, this would seem the wisest practice. In a normal thriving infant in the UK, my experience is that continuation of breast/milk feeding increases the volume of liquid stools and enhances the risk of developing transient lactose/milk intolerance, therefore altering the balance in favour of a different practice. There is good evidence that a significant number of infants, even after mild diarrhoea, show damage to the small intestinal mucosa. Subsequent transient lactose, cows' milk protein and even gluten intolerance may ensue.

My approach attempts to minimize symptoms and complications and ideally I use oral rehydrating solutions, withdrawing milk (breast/bottle) for 24 hours. In an infant of this age I would regrade the feeds in 24 h sequences: no milk; ¼ strength; ½ strength etc. I add 5 g (1 level teaspoonful) of pure glucose powder to each 100 ml of ¼ strength and ½ strength milk, to increase calorie intake. This mother would probably succeed with 'spooned' liquid – not as slow as it seems for an experienced mother. She would need a breast pump to evacuate the milk for regrading and ensure lactation continues. If this really were impossible I would continue breast-feeding and try some spooned oral rehydrating fluid as 'extra' after each feed. An older infant (e.g. 4 months) would certainly manage a spoon and milk can be substituted by a range of non-provocative calories to compensate, e.g. chicken, rice, potato, apple, etc., all puréed with boiled water. It is important to remember that prolonged and profuse diarrhoea worries mothers a great deal (but rarely bothers research workers) and causes some very excoriated buttocks at minimum!

Question 70. Encopresis or constipation?

How would you differentiate between encopresis and constipation in a child of 6 years with soiling but with no apparent psychological disturbance? Are laxatives effective in the treatment of encopresis?

It depends what you mean by encopresis. . . and constipation!

Constipation implies symptoms and upset for the child and does not mean merely the character of the stool. I use the word 'encopresis' as synonymous with soiling in a child, approximately 3 years or older, who should be continent of stool. Some reserve the word 'encopresis' for normal stools released/placed in abnormal places – a clear disturbance of psychological origin.

You must always detail the history of the child's defecation. Has he always soiled (primary encopresis) or has he had a period of success and then relapsed (secondary encopresis)? Without obvious psychological factors this case is much more likely to be primary, probably a failure to learn. Are the stools normal or abnormal? Normal stools would favour the 'failure to learn' origins. Massive hard stools with or without foul smelling, dark liquid overflow suggests 'retention with overflow'. Examine the abdomen. Are there rocks to confirm the latter? If not, liquid stools suggests diarrhoea, e.g. colitis, or bulky stools coeliac disease with secondary soiling. The algorithm, Figure 9, may help you through the major causes.

Constipation (symptomatic delayed passage of stool) without soiling rarely occurs secondary to other illness. At the age of 6 years, few should have escaped earlier recognition:

• Intercurrent infection with dehydration.
• Hypokalaemia complicating diarrhoea.
• Hypothyroidism.

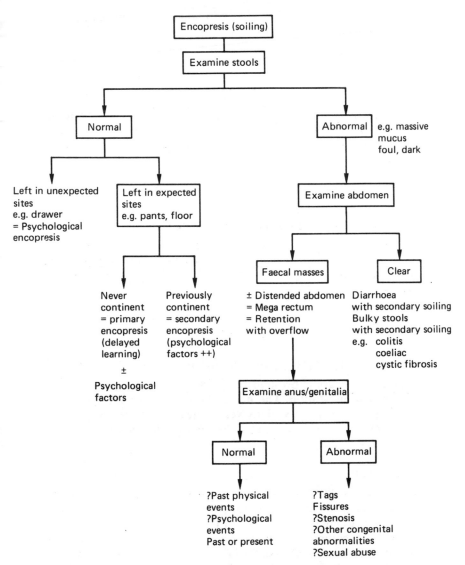

Figure 9 Causes of encopresis

- Neurological disease especially of the spinal cord or cerebral palsy.
- Metabolic disease, e.g. hyperparathyroidism; renal tubular acidosis.
- Lead poisoning.
- Gastro-intestinal disease, e.g. coeliac, cystic fibrosis.

Treatment should be individually planned according to cause, with enhancement of normal physiological processes wherever possible, e.g. increasing fluids, dietary fibre, encouraging good toilet routines. Laxatives are useful for:

- Keeping stools soft – *bulk laxatives* – trap water, e.g. methyl cellulose and lactulose, reducing the ability to withhold.
- Dispersing retained stool – *faecal softeners* – e.g. Docusate (Dioctyl) emulsifying effect on large faecal masses.
- Hastening passage – *stimulant laxatives* – e.g. Senna or Bisacodyl (Dulcolax), once large retained stools cleared. In combination with softener, this will help clear the rectum and reduce distension. May be needed for a prolonged period.

Suppositories and enemas should be avoided or limited to a minimum. Evacuation under anaesthesia is often preferred in desperate situations, where starting 'afresh' is necessary before laxatives are effective.

Most situations require a careful combination of counselling or behavioural modification techniques and appropriate laxative medication for shorter or longer periods.

Question 71. 'He's got worms again!'

A child of 7 years is brought to the doctor – yet again – with a threadworm infestation. The doctor looks through the notes and finds that he has used various vermicides in the past on at least five separate occasions. What is he, or the child's parents, most likely doing wrong?

Using a feather duster instead of a sledgehammer.

Here are my anecdotal experiences:

- *Thumbsuckers* – incurable vectors – but I may buy a long remission by my 'blitzkrieg' approach (see infra).
- *Baths* – communal, with flannels and sponges, plastic menageries and naval bases – don't help. While treating, lose the expendable and leave the heirlooms in a bucket of disinfectant (vinegarized water works well).
- *Sleuth* – for unexpected practices, e.g. all the children's bottoms being washed with the same cloth/flannel after defecation.
- *Do unto others* – taste the antihelminth you prescribe and record your likely 'compliance' score.

I use Mebendazole tablets only – 100 mg (½ tablet, 50 mg, for the under 3s and 1 tablet, 100 mg, for everyone else). The tablets are fairly tasteless and can be crushed in a drink for the younger ones. I try to decide who might be heavily infected (symptomatic) i.e. complaining of recurrent nocturnal/anal/vulval pain and/or pruritus.

		←		Day			→
		1	2	3	4	5	6–13	14
<3 Years	Itchy anus/vulva	½	½	½	½	½	0	½
<3 Years	Asymptomatic	½	0	0	0	0	0	½
>3 Years	Itchy anus/vulva	1	1	1	1	1	0	1
>3 Years	Asymptomatic	1	0	0	0	0	0	1

Ensure you include the whole human population living in the house.

I also recommend that all bed linen and pyjamas of infected individuals are left to soak in a bucket of vinegarized water overnight and then washed in a washing machine the next day. This should reduce re-infection chances considerably.

Question 72. Hiatus hernia in infancy

A child of 3 months is brought to the doctor by a distraught mother. The child seems quite well but the mother says that half an hour after being fed he begins to scream, apparently with pain, in the most inconsolable fashion, for about half an hour. The doctor can find no abnormality. The mother says that her friend's baby with similar symptoms was diagnosed by a paediatrician as having a hiatus hernia. Would this story be typical? Would it be worth trying a small amount of H_2 antagonist before resorting to a barium meal?

This story, without vomiting, is not typical. I would try some Gaviscon but not an H_2 antagonist without proof of reflux.

Hiatus hernia is an uncommon condition in infancy, though increased use of pH-monitoring by probe – preferable to X-ray – has shown that gastro-oesophageal reflux (GOR) is not.

GOR can present in a number of ways:

• Gastro-intestinal – vomiting (after and between feeds), haematemesis, failure to thrive, abdominal and/or chest pain, dysphagia, anaemia.
• Respiratory – recurrent chest infection (especially aspiration into lower lobes), recurrent wheeze (especially in an under 6 months child with night-time vomiting), apnoeic spells including near-miss cot death, unexplained choking spells.

- Neurological – unexplained irritability, seizure-like periods around feed times.

It must be differentiated from atypical 3-month colic, cow's milk allergy, congenital intestinal abnormalities and congenital heart disease, the symptoms of which may be provoked by eating.

I would not consider this infant's symptoms to be the usual manifestation of GOR. Vomiting is far more frequently the indicator, especially associated with prolonged crying after the vomit and particularly if 'coffee-grounds' or blood are seen in the vomitus. Low birthweight infants subjected to intensive care (ventilation) frequently present with respiratory manifestations with or without a pattern of vomiting.

Having considered and clinically excluded rarities, e.g. ultrasound and a straight X-ray of abdomen, it would not be amiss to try:

- Infant Gaviscon 1 sachet in each feed if bottle fed or made up with 15 ml water and given after breast feeds.

   plus

- Carobel to thicken feeds

I would be very loathe to empirically use H_2 antagonists; or cisapride without proving the presence of significant GOR by pH studies.

Question 73. Relieving colic

In the past it has been the practice of many doctors to give 'colicky' babies dicyclomine syrup – not least as a placebo for the mother. This medication is now contraindicated in young infants. Faced with such a problem now, is there any other substance that could be recommended that might, at least in part, bring relief to child and mother... and doctor?

Colic, to some degree, is the norm. Treatment may largely depend on the family's ability to cope with it.

The classic presentation of 3-month colic is appearance in the first week or two of life, when, between 18.00 and 22.00 hours, some 30 minutes after the evening feed, the infant screams blue-facedly, pulls up his/her legs and often passes flatus up and down with loud rumblings (borborygmi) audible in the abdomen and with periods of quiet or sleep between pains. This may merge into a pattern of crying with colicky like pains throughout the day and night. I believe that 3-month colic is a result of the baby adopting his/her own diurnal and circadian rhythms as opposed to the intrauterine, maternal rhythms enjoyed by the fetus. In this sense a degree of 'colic' is to be expected in every baby.

The medical role is:

- To exclude alternative (disease) explanations.
- To help the family understand how such pain can be benign and thereby reassure.
- To support the family through this exhausting time by sharing the particular homespun hypothesis (and/or placebo) that you think can safely help. Colic can produce many levels of difficulty and the family predicaments that go with it can be just as variable – weaving a variety of need for medication or alternative support:

I may work through:

- Activated dimethicone. Infacol, 0.5 ml contains 20 mg, given before feeds, especially those which seem to precede the colic.
- Occasionally, lactose-free/cow's-milk-protein-free milk, if this is a formula fed baby with a strong family history of allergy/food intolerance. A short trial, easy at this age, should show quick and dramatic response or be abandoned. Reducing cow's milk and occasionally other allergens in the diet of a breast-fed mother can be tried, but with careful attention to mother's nutritional needs.
- Chloral hydrate 15–30 mg/kg per dose given 15 minutes before the provocative feed/feeds, no more frequently than 8-hourly may damp down the severity of the colic.
- Trimeprazine 2–3 mg/kg per dose given 1 hour before usual onset or worst time of day may act similarly to chloral in damping down severity of response. I only use these latter approaches to buy a short period of respite for exhausted parents and I constantly push for weaning off or withholding.
- Admission to the paediatric ward. One or two nights sleep for parents, using skilled 'babysitters' who can observe and sometimes suggest remedies, may break the pattern of 'hell' where all symptoms lose their perspective.

Question 74. Abdominal pain of childhood. How much investigation?

For several months a girl of 6 years has been backwards and forwards to the GP with abdominal pain. Both full blood count and urine tests are normal. There are no abnormal physical signs.

The child is eating well and has not lost weight. There is a possibility of bullying at school though the child denies this. The doctor diagnoses 'abdominal pain of childhood'. Can such a diagnosis be made safely without further investigation? How long should a doctor leave it before something else (What?) is done?

The condition has a very recognizable profile. Ninety-five per cent of the children affected have no underlying physical pathology.

Serious readers will I hope turn to the writings of the late John Apley for the full answer to this question. Read his collected papers (1987) to savour his infinite wisdom on all aspects of recurrent abdominal pain (RAP) in childhood, but better still the broad exciting canvas of his paediatric art. My experience has never been able to contradict his teachings:

- He studied 1000 children and followed some of them for more than 2 decades.
- At least three bouts of pain, severe enough to affect activity, over a period not less than 3 months and having been present the year of the study constituted his criteria.
- The incidence was about 1 in 10 for all children from the age of 5 years with a high peak in girls aged 9 years (up to 1 in 4).
- *Less than 5%* of the affected children had evidence of organic disease and half of these were urinary tract infections.
- There was a high incidence of RAP in the family (First degree relatives) – 46% (as opposed to only 8% in controls) – what he describes as 'painful families'.
- *The further the localization of abdominal pain from the umbilicus the more likely is there to be underlying disease* is his historic aphorism (or Apleyism). Two-thirds felt pain at or around the umbilicus.
- Apart from localization, no other characterization of the pain helped discriminate organic from non-organic cases (e.g. severity, frequency, night pain, vomiting and associated factors).
- He produced a clinical profile of 'the whole child' who had

  a) A history of recurrent symptoms often including limb pains and headaches.
  b) A slightly underweight child.
  c) A timid, anxious and excessively conscientious personality.
  d) A pattern of emotional disturbances, e.g. enuresis, nightmares and sleep problems, appetite difficulties.
  e) A 'whole family' who also had higher incidence of recurrent pains and nervous disorders.

- Apley used 'informal psychotherapy' with considerable success and formulated a conceptual model of the many factors promoting psychosomatic illness.

In summary, the high incidence of RAP, the typical history (which must be meticulously combed through), the complete absence of clinical signs (methodically completed) with positive evidence of family pattern or emotional upheaval (the bullying in this case), and assurance that the urine is clear, leaves no doubt about the diagnosis and does not warrant any further testing.

I rarely seek a full blood count, but slightly more often use an ultrasound of the abdomen in severe, atypical pains (Apley missed one case with ovarian cysts – but did not have ultrasound at his disposal!). It is vital to reassure (the careful history and examination goes a long way towards that) and to reassure *with explanation*. I use the analogy of an adult's fear at his/her wedding or interview for a vital job and the indisputable physical response of, e.g. frequency of micturition, or frequent loose stool or sweating and palpitations, that disappear when the 'stress' is over.

This illustrates to most, including the child, the part the mind plays over the body, i.e. an attempt to conceptualize psychosomatic symptoms. I also ensure that an illustration of a child's fears or anxieties destroys any ideas that children 'don't have worries', e.g. the demands of school for the first time, the acted out behaviour of other children, the scare stories of death. The child's turmoils will not be patently obvious or directly related to the pain (but often are when you reach the true events). Knowledge of the family and child may indicate a need for more intensive explanation or help for serious emotional problems, but the vast majority can be passed back to capable parents once their minds are open to the real situation and relieved of the 'physical' fear. I would always wish to review that symptoms have improved – not too soon to signal doubt – but, say, 3 months to ensure success.

Failure to respond should lead to more 'structured' psychosomatic investigation as Apley warns that untreated 'little belly achers grow up to be big belly achers'.

Question 75.   When should a normal diet restart with gastroenteritis?

A child of 18 months develops diarrhoea. The GP prescribes rehydrating medicine and reassures the mother. The child is not ill but the diarrhoea continues. Three days later a stool sample is sent to the laboratory. The mother continues with clear fluids but the child begins to lose weight. Three days later the pathology laboratory, reports a rotavirus infection. Though not acutely ill the child continues with diarrhoea and loss of weight. What can

be done? Is it harmful to reintroduce solids to a hungry child with persistent diarrhoea?

You must increase the intake of calories.

As has been said in Question 69, rotavirus is the commonest cause of gastroenteritis in children in the UK. There is, however, a different situation here. At this later age the child's diet is more comprehensive, giving a wider choice than just the milk or clear fluid available to the young infant. Indeed, in the treatment of this toddler's diarrhoea, milk is more troublesome.

It is essential to rehydrate with oral fluids. A lot of 18-month children refuse 'salty' prepared electrolyte solutions and resorting to the child's favourite 'clear fluid' is acceptable, e.g. Ribena, apple juice, etc. Never use these drinks ice-cold as this only increases peristalsis. Although many would counsel continuation of normal diet, I would not in the generally well nourished UK inhabitant. Milk products (due to lactose) are likely to prolong and aggravate the diarrhoea and, in a few cases, can produce severe secondary intolerance with vomiting, etc.

At 18 months I advise staying off milk until all diarrhoea has gone, 1–2 weeks if necessary but IT IS VITAL TO SUBSTITUTE ADEQUATE CALORIES. After 24 hours of clear fluids I will advise rice, potato, chicken, fruit and vegetables, in fact, anything but milk products (I would also exclude wheat in the worst cases). Should the diarrhoea persist beyond 2 weeks, supplements of calcium and vitamins can be added.

Feeding

Question 76. The vegan baby

The mother of a 1-year-old child tells her family doctor that the whole family, including the baby, are on a vegan diet, the result of her recent conversion by a television programme. How much harm, if any, could this cause to a developing baby? Should omnivorous diets be encouraged for babies and toddlers?

The more restricted the diet, the more danger there is of deficiencies, and the more supplements have to be given.

Appreciating a rich variety of foods is likely to benefit children and avoid deficiencies of minor nutrients. Certain ethnic and religious cultures use food as symbolic of self-meaning and discipline. Unusual, sometimes bizarre and restrictive, diets may produce risks for children.

Vegetarian diets can vary from the partial vegetarian (avoiding red meat) right through to the vegan diet (avoiding all animal products including milk and eggs). The problems facing a small child fed a strict vegetarian diet are:

- Insufficient calories – plant food is low in calories and this must be made up for by more frequent feeding and the addition of vegetable fats and oils.
- Insufficient high class protein – there is variable amino acid content in plant protein and the protein can be of low biological value. The most widely used plant proteins are the pulses and legumes which can be indigestible for the small child. Eggs and milk would, be a natural source but are excluded for the vegan. Pulses etc. may need to be ground up.
- Insufficient minerals – the best source of iron is meat. From vegetables its absorption is unpredictable and needs a plentiful supply of ascorbic acid. Dark green vegetables contain more iron. Soya based 'milks' have added iron, calcium and vitamins.
- Vitamin supplements have to be given as there is very little vitamin D and vitamin B12 in non-animal products. Yeast can provide riboflavin, etc.

It can be seen that a considerable knowledge of nutrition will be needed to provide an adequate diet for a rapidly growing child. A larger bulk of food is required (remember, grazing, i.e. vegetarian animals, have to spend half their life eating), and there can be a danger of aspiration or choking, in young children, on nuts, seeds, etc.

Traditional methods of cooking in a culture may be changed, and devalued, when moved to another country. If milk is allowed its bulk may diminish the intake of other foods. Growth must be monitored closely. Soy-based formula, vitamin and mineral supplements must come from a reliable source. Many health food shops sell products with no professional supervision to monitor suitability or balance or source.

We should not attempt to overturn or be dismissive of tradition or personal choice, but scientifically advise and offer professional support to ensure safe and adequate nutrition.

Question 77.   How often is soya justified?

At the onset of relatively minor abdominal and feeding upsets some mothers are happy to change the baby over to one of the soya based 'milks'. Is the successful outcome of their manoeuvre probably more apparent than real? Is it often really justified or are the mothers making a rod for their own backs... 'He mustn't have any kind of dairy products!'

Only 1 in 20 infants have any genuine degree of cow's milk allergy (CMA), mostly minor. An 'allergic' status can be very demanding.

The underlying question is which infants have a high possibility of having CMA or cow's milk protein intolerance. There is a further subdivision:

- Indirect effect – the entirely breast-fed infant receiving allergens through mother's diet, i.e. transmitted via breast milk.
- Direct effect – the infant being supplemented with, complemented with, or entirely formula fed.

The overall incidence of CMA has been projected to be about 5% of the population under 1 year of age. Severe reactions to milk ingestion have been identified in some 1 in 4 (25%) of all proven CMA cases, leaving 3 in 4 (of 5%), i.e. nearly 4 cases in every 100 infants, who may have relatively mild symptomatology, such as colic, loose stools, rashes, eczema, irritability and poor weight gain (see Table 7).

Many mothers are attempting an exclusion diet but are unaware of the pitfalls. Doctors (some) would prefer a more rigorous adherence to academic principles *that few of us can live by*.

It would be preferable to:

- Have a skin test – not absolute by any means, but can be a point in favour. All other tests in current clinical use are no more sensitive and a lot more expensive, e.g. radio-allergoabsorbent test (RAST) (in CMA at least).

Table 7. Clinical features of 100 infants with proved cow's milk allergy

Clinical features[a]	Incidence
Gastrointestinal	
Vomiting	41
Diarrhoea	48
Colic	14
Colitis[b]	4
Functional intestinal obstruction[b]	3
Generalized anaphylaxis[b]	
Stridor, collapse	2
Dermatological features	
Urticaria (general)	10
Angioedema	13
Circumoral lesions	26
Morbilliform eruptions	6
Eczema	13
Perianal eruptions	1
Respiratory	
Stridor (recurrent)	4
Rhinitis	21
Cough, wheeze	29
Tachypnoea	1
Nervous system	
Irritability[b]	40
Syncope–collapse alone[b]	12
Convulsions[b]	2
Other manifestations	
Anaemia[b]	2
Osteoporosis[b]	1
Severe failure to thrive[c]	22
Gross gastroesophageal reflux (radiological)[b]	6

[a] All symptoms elicited by challenge unless otherwise indicated.
[b] Features attributed to milk ingestion prior to formal challenge.
[c] Weight <3rd percentile.
From David, T.J. (1991) *Recent Advances in Paediatrics*, p. 188, Edinburgh: Churchill Livingstone

- Implement a trial off all cow's milk for 6 weeks, with resolution of symptoms, and
- Show on re-introduction (challenge) of cow's milk formula that symptoms return.

In the young infant (under 6 months) such an approach is easily handled, and safe. Mothers need to be reminded to avoid cow's milk products in any solids they may wish to introduce during the trial period – using the substituted milk for cereals, etc.

It must be warned that quite a high percentage of infants with CMA have hypersensitivity to other foods, including soy protein. I prefer to opt for an 'elemental' substitute such as Prejomin or Pregestimil. Although more expensive (and there is a need to slowly regrade onto such a formula), a trial period is achieved without wondering if there might be a complicating soy hypersensitivity issue. I would similarly avoid (taking out or not adding in) potential confusers such as wheat/egg/lactose (especially in medicines). I would not include infants with symptoms starting after 6 months of unproblematic cow's milk formula feeding. Hopefully breast-feeding is still and will remain the usual form of infant feeding, although the drop-out rate at 6 weeks is still alarmingly high. The decision to exclude cow's milk from the mother's own diet is much more difficult and I would seek more exacting reasons, e.g. strong family history of allergy; severity of symptoms etc. I would then ensure that a mother determined to try, or where clinically indicated, should have careful dietary guidance, especially regarding calcium, and vitamin needs.

Question 78. The fish finger diet. Are vitamins needed?

A GP is informed by the worried parents of a 4-year-old that their robust and fit-looking son exists 'entirely on fish fingers, crisps, chocolate and ice-cream, Doctor', eschewing all other foods. Should more control be exerted over the child in spite of the mother's protestations that she has 'tried and tried'? Should vitamin supplements be given? Are vitamin supplements ever, indeed, needed by normal children or is their prescription merely a placebo for the parents?

Children tend to eat what they fancy. A proper dose of vitamin supplement is a good safety net.

It sounds like a typical medical house officer's diet to me! Perhaps the analogy should not end there. A good training consists of setting clear goals in a language appropriate to degree of understanding. Next, good models are demonstrated (one's own behaviour) and all good efforts are encouraged and rewarded. Like SHOs, 4-year-olds are highly intelligent, energetic, but frantically busy people.....in the main!

I would stick to a few basic rules (Question 80) but strongly advise against intimidatory practices, as resentment and sabotage might result. I often ask a parent to supply a diary of a week's intake by the child, in quality and quantity. A dietitian can analyse, often by pressing the computer buttons, the appropriate properties of the nutrition eaten. Suggestions regarding vital supplements can then be decided, e.g. marmite flavoured crisps. There is a lot of good protein in fish fingers and the likely marginal zones will be in minerals (calcium, iron) and vitamins (Table 8).

Table 8. Recommended daily intake for 4 year old

Water soluble vitamins

Thiamine (B1)	Riboflavin	Niacin	B$_6$(pyridoxine)	B$_{12}$	Vit. C	Folic acid
0.9 mg	1.0 mg	11 mg	1.6 mg	1.5 µg	50 mg	100–300 µg

Fat soluble vitamins

Vit. A	Vit. D	Vit. E
500 µg	10 µg	6 mg
(retinol)	1 µg = 40 IU	α-Tocopherol

Minerals

Iron	Zinc	Copper	Calcium	Fluoride
7 mg	10 mg	2 mg	400–800 mg	1.0 mg
				IF <1ppm in H$_2$O

A recent study from our community showed disturbing gaps in vitamin knowledge within families with reference to children under 5 years.

- 22% taking an incorrect dosage (fortunately too little, but we have written up severe overdosages too).
- 45% not taking any at all.
- 35% not knowing when to stop supplementation.
  Professional supervision seemed very flimsy.

The recommended dosages of vitamins at various ages are given in Table 8.

In the main, children in the UK are fed minimal or suboptimal levels of vitamins, and with recent studies suggesting these may influence children's scholastic performance, I would counsel parents to give added supplements. They need written guidance for the correct dosage and when to change dosage or stop. Preparations should be bought from community health clinics or from pharmacies and not health food shops where there are many ill-balanced and inappropriate alternatives.

Question 79. Hungry at 4 weeks. Are solids needed?

A baby boy of 4 weeks is very hungry indeed. The mother tells the doctor that the only way she has been able to satisfy him is by giving him solids. Under what age would you consider it inadvisable to give solids in any circumstances?

Solids at 4 weeks are generally not a good idea. Four months is a more suitable time. 'Hungry' might result from underfeeding or might represent something else entirely.

In the presence of gastro-intestinal reflux we often thicken feeds at this age. Some brain-injured babies with incoordinate swallowing manage solids better than liquids. Babies with severe cardiac problems may need extra calories in solid form to compensate for limitations on fluid intake. These are examples of instances where solids at a very early age overcome fairly dire, yet uncommon, predicaments.

This is a far cry from colluding with such an approach for normal babies. I would reaffirm that the corporate wisdom suggests introduction of solids at about 4 months of age, based on knowledge of the infant's limitations in coping with solute loads until the kidneys have 'matured'. I would never be dogmatic, but informative, and most importantly I would check the history and the child, including measurements and observing a feed, to ensure I did not miss a better explanation for the infant's supposed hunger:

- If breast fed, with a discrepancy in weight for length and head circumference, and frequent green stools, it might indicate that breast milk production is falling behind – 4–6 weeks being a common water shed – and that the baby is, indeed hungry. There are other alternatives to solids that may be used.
- If formula fed, improper reconstitution of feed, incorrect volume for expected (not actual) weight, cow's milk allergy, might all lead to a 'crying' infant.
- The pattern of hunger might follow 3-month colic responses where feeding may diminish crying temporarily (see Colic, Question 73).
- The vast majority of such babies are '*overactive*' infants (not to be confused with hyperactivity).

These overactive infants appear more wakeful and alert from the moment of birth, with big swings in their behaviour from deep sleep to wakefulness and crying, rather than going through a gradual transition. They are restless, constantly moving when awake unless 'engaged' in something interesting. They cry a lot, gulp food, suck anything, are often colicky and although exciting, the babies are exhausting to care for. This is a behavioural pattern, not a disease, and affects some 25% of normal infants. All pressurize the unwary parents (and doctors). Who would not assume hunger in such babies? Who would not want to try food as a panacea?

Such infants are readily spotted if you watch them feed and have an observation session. For further reading see, 'Infants and Mothers' by T.B. Brazelton, Hutchinson 1972.

My final advice is to share your knowledge and experience with parents, but do not be prescriptive.

Question 80.   The fat toddler and dieting

A girl of 3 years is very fat. Both mother and father are fat. At this age would your aim be to maintain the child at her present weight and let natural development thin her down, or would you take active steps to make her lose weight? Is there an age below which you would not advise weight reduction? Are there any general guide lines on dieting small children?

Fat toddlers usually thin down by the age of 5 years but most, with this little girl's history, unmanaged, become permanently fat again later.

If you compared two obese infants, one having obese parents, the other not, the former will have 6 times more chance of becoming an obese child. Yet relatively few infants continue their fatness up to 5 years of age, so refattening may develop at any time and continue into adult life. It would be helpful to know the previous dynamics of the 3-year-old as she may just be 'on the way down'. Not all the issues regarding the risks of childhood obesity are clear, but if only 10% persist through to adulthood, I would want to turn the tide as soon as possible. But beware:

* Failure rate is depressingly high.
* Severe curtailment of nutrition in a rapidly growing child may deplete other tissues than fat.

Therefore DRIVE THE FAMILY MAD! (Motivation, Activity, Diet).

M is for Motivation:

* Make sure, and reassure, that no illness is missed. The triad of fatness, shortness and developmental slowness, particularly, may point to dysmorphic syndromes like Prader–Willi or Lawrence–Moon–Biedl, or endocrine disorders such as hypothyroidism or pseudohypoparathyroidism. A fat 3-year-

old, rather unusual in my experience, deserves particular care here. Anything approaching a 'Pickwickian syndrome' where obesity interferes with ventilation, leading to CO_2 retention and somnolence, requires drastic action.

- Educate on the obesity-related diseases of adulthood.
- Explain that holding weight steady, in a rapidly growing child, will achieve as much as weight loss at this stage. Recommend 'Looking to make kids slim!' by A. Ellis, which is a user-friendly book.
- Encourage early entry into a well-briefed, supportive nursery or play group to distance the child from larder or 'wavering' parent.

A is for Activity:

- Walking everywhere, forgetting the car, maybe buying a dog.
- Swimming pool parties, not videos.
- Join all the tumbletots, music and movement, aerobics, fun runs and adventure playground activities. Get the whole family exercising.

D is for Diet:

- Keep a diary of all items eaten.
- Ban from house sweets, crisps, biscuits, cakes and ice-cream. Most of all ban sweet 'energy-giving' drinks. A can of cola contains 7 teaspoonfuls of sugar, one of the highly advertised 'sports drinks' contains 12 spoonfuls of sugar in one can. Many children will drink two cans at a sitting. Low calorie drinks will resist peer pressure.
- Eliminate snacks. Distract with activity.
- Reduce all sugars and fats.
- In dire circumstances a yet stricter diet will be needed. Consult the dietician. Defining obesity is very difficult at this age. A rule of thumb is 20% above average weight for age, sex and height and a 1 inch skin fold pinched over triceps, lower end of scapula or supra-iliac region.

Question 81. 'E-itis'

A child of 4 years is irritable, uncooperative and generally bad-tempered. His 9-year-old sister is attending the child psychologist for behavioural problems. The mother is convinced that the smaller child is suffering from the effects of food additives and asks how to put the child on an exclusion diet. How frequently are children really affected by 'E's – artificial colours, preservatives, etc. – and how often is it that they are just irritable, unco-

operative and generally bad-tempered from having a mother who won't let them eat sweets and crisps and a maladjusted sister who thumps them when Mum isn't looking?

Behavioural problems are extremely common, genuine 'E' sensitivity problems are not.

W.S. Gilbert, were he alive, would find this an ideal subject for ridiculing the medical profession – perhaps calling it 'Rudd-E-gore' (or doctors curse). Some observations:

- *A hyperkinetic syndrome* exists, in which the child displays unending restlessness, impulsiveness, rapid mood swings, butterfly concentration, distractibility, poor sleeping pattern and often with aggressiveness, bad behaviour, clumsiness and learning difficulties. Seen 4 times more often in boys, it has been surveyed as occurring in 1 in 1000 children in the UK (but 30 in 1000 in the USA). Modern parlance calls this an attention deficit disorder or syndrome (ADD or ADS).
- *Allergic responses* such as angio-oedema, urticaria and asthma have been clearly described, mostly as immediate-type IgE reactions to chemicals which are known artificial additives, e.g. tartrazine (E102), benzoate (E211). A multicentre study in the UK reported in 1987 estimated a prevalence of 0.01–0.23% (up to 2.3 per 1000) for food additive intolerance in general.
- *Behaviour problems* (emotional and conduct) are extremely common, perhaps involving up to 10% of all children, and the symptoms have a biological continuum with those described in ADD. Many factors, such as those social, economic and neurodevelopmental, play a significant part in their causation.

The difficulties arise where an attempt is made to clinically relate all manner of behavioural responses to all manner of food additives. Where an acute allergic response can be observed, it can be relatively easy to scientifically appraise. But delayed (late) allergic responses which we know exist, e.g. in asthma, are almost impossible to prove beyond doubt by ingestion.

What is the doctor to do?

- He should adhere to medical science and explain that 'quick-fix' approaches to such problems are not available.
- It makes good sense to avoid unnecessary junk food with pointless pretty colours. But it is invidious to evaluate the philosophy and economics of good versus bad food.
- Extremely difficult predicaments warrant an open-minded approach with devoted search of detail, attempting to assess important contributive elements and evaluate any potential for change:

(a) A strong family history of allergy especially to some foods.
(b) A previous history of confirmed allergy in the child in earlier years, e.g. eczema or gastro-intestinal upset.
(c) Early schooling or nursery to remove the child from sweets, crisps and a bad tempered mother and sister, for long enough periods for everyone to feel better (except perhaps teacher!)
(d) The behavioural therapist may have a colleague running a mother–child interaction group where observation of the problem might shed light on the dynamics.
(e) A limited, structured elimination diet, supervised by a dietitian, can be tried based on parental hunches. Parents should be dissuaded from 'doing it alone' because of the real dangers of hypoallergenic diets. There can be a fine line between allergy obsession and abuse of the child.
(f) Modern methods of videoing disturbed behaviour as a baseline for 'double-blind' challenging may prove a way forward.

I am not convinced dietary factors play an important role in any but a tiny number of behavioural situations. I am not convinced parents can 'deliver' an objective trial in such difficult 4-year-olds. I am convinced such problems must be listened to, thought about and constructively dealt with.

'My name is John Wellington Wells! I'm a dealer in magic and spells'.

Question 82.   Feeds taken – no weight gain

A baby of 6 weeks is referred to the doctor by a health visitor because there has been no increase in weight for 3 weeks. The baby is bottle fed by an intelligent mother. There are no abnormal physical findings. How should the doctor proceed?

Remembering that the cause might be pathological, genetic or simply a case of under-feeding.

This is a tricky problem and I would want to see all the previous measurements, including those of length and head circumference. Some babies with excellent fetal growth need to drop across the percentile to reach their true (genetic) tramline which may be lower, i.e. fetal growth and initial post-natal growth can change gear in later infancy. Head circumference and length might slow down too in proportion to weight slowing.

I would also:

- Recalculate the daily intake relative to the expected (as opposed to actual weight). Thus a small for dates baby, e.g. 3 kg at 6 weeks needs 150 ml/kg per day calculated on 4 kg not 3 kg, in order to gain satisfactorily, i.e. 600 ml/day not 450 ml. The baby may simply not be getting enough to eat!
- Watch the baby feed – you will see if sucking is vigorous or the baby lethargic, breathless or feeble (health visitors are invaluable here.)
- Look at (and smell) the infant's stool – the dark green, slightly mucousy stool of starvation or the malodorous, greasy, bulky pervasive stool of cystic fibrosis could be instant indicators.

Without a good explanation a clean catch urine must be cultured. Twenty-four or 48 hours with an experienced paediatric sister (preferably one who works in the community and visits home) or else a short ward admission must be the next stage in assessment.

Skin

Question 83. Antibiotics for eczema

A GP is treating a little boy of 3 years with severe eczema. On two occasions within 3 or 4 months of each other the child has a throat infection for which the doctor prescribes an antibiotic. On each occasion the eczema seems to become much less severe. Is it most likely coincidental?

No.

Some of the greatest discoveries in medicine were made by persons not prepared to accept coincidence. I do not think there is a Nobel prize in the offing for realizing an explanation here. *Staphylococcus, Streptococcus* and *Haemophilus* can all too frequently be isolated from the lesions of severe (especially weeping) eczema. Topical preparations combining antibiotics and steroids may heal while steroid alone may worsen a severe exacerbation of eczema. Someone prescribing penicillin, erythromycin or a broader spectrum cephalosporin for a sore throat (presumed or proved) should not be surprised if the child's severe weeping eczema dramatically improves without any other manipulation of skin management.

Many dermatologists and paediatricians when confronted with a child with an acute exacerbation of eczema, after taking the appropriate swabs, will give a course of oral antibiotics at the outset. Flucloxacillin or erythromycin are often used in these circumstances. There would be little harm in the family doctor trying such a manoeuvre even without the benefit of microbiological confirmation.

Question 84. Is hydrocortisone 1% harmful?

A breast-fed baby of 3 months has developed quite marked eczema of body and face. Is the use of hydrocortisone cream or ointment justified in all areas? If so, in what strength and how often... and for how long?

Hydrocortisone 1% is very safe.

Severe eczema in a young infant is a frightening and demoralizing disease for a family to endure, especially as the parents almost certainly have been told, or read, it is rare or uncommon in breast-fed infants. It is a delicate juggling act to convince them of the need for steroids (which they also have been told, or read, are mainly evil). It may need a trial of less effective measures first, leaving the doctor on a hiding to nothing, as lack of instant success may mean the parents hastily resort to 'alternative medicines'. Hordes of these exist, employing media skills with which scientific medicine is neither able, nor allowed to compete. Effective communication and education is difficult within a scenario of stress. Provided I can convince the parents of my best intentions, I would use hydrocortisone early.

Unless the eczema is weeping, ointment is superior to cream. It is now clear that less than 1% hydrocortisone is ineffective and 1% will never harm, however much is used anywhere on the body. Used three times a day with other measures it is rarely necessary to ascend to higher potency steroid strength. The maxim 'lowest effective potency for least time' must be respected.

Question 85. Non-steroid preparations for eczema

A doctor is faced with a 4-month child new to the list. Although breast-fed, she has eczema and the only treatment previously given has been a steroid cream. What else might be of help?

A variety of measures and some reassessment.
Amongst the measures I would suggest trying are:

- A careful trawl through possible new allergens introduced, mostly unwittingly, at a time of exacerbating skin disease, e.g. new dietary fads (given to mother or child) especially from health food shops; medications; washing materials; clothing, e.g. wool.
- Frequent cleansing in baths neither hot nor prolonged, using emollient instead of soap.
- Potassium permanganate baths (Permitabs – 1 tablet in 4 litres of water, 0.01% solution) rapidly help heal infected eczema, especially from the waist down, even if it ruins the whisper apricot bathware (use an old plastic bowl).
- Oral antibiotics and even steroid with topical antibiotic (see Question 83).
- Appropriate addition of coal tar (anti-inflammatory antipruritic and keratolytic), calamine (antipruritic) urea, fossil fish oil (icthamol), perhaps in the form of impregnated bandages.
- Emollients.
- Antipruritic e.g. Trimeprazine 2 mg/kg if severe itching.

Bath emollients which eliminate the need for soap must be easy
to use (ung. emulsificans has to be melted in a small amount of
very hot water in order to disperse – very user unfriendly,
however cheap). Creaming with moisturizers (emollient) is easiest
after a bath, but in order to instil as a reflex response at all other
times the infant seems uncomfortable itchy and dry, should be in
a ready to hand dispenser and acceptable to the parent's 'taste'.
Although I explore Unguentum Merck and Diprobase as my
current firsts, I list several others for the parents to experiment
with – two preparations at a time – comparing one side of the
infant's body with the other.

A strongly correlating change in severity of eczema with a clear
'adventure' in mother's diet would certainly be worth pursuing
but I am loathe to manipulate the mother's nutrition in a blind
attempt. At this baby's age, I would be prepared, with expert
dietary assistance, to have a trial of elimination of cow's milk, egg
and possibly wheat in the mother's diet provided the severity of
disease warrants such action, that the parents contract to cease
after 6 weeks if no clear advantage ensues, and that the dietitian's
rules obtain with regard to supplementary replacement.

Question 86. Look carefully at nappy rash

**A child of 4 months has severe nappy rash which resolves rapidly
with a nystatin/hydrocortisone cream. Within a few days of
stopping the treatment the rash returns. The mother uses it again
with the same series of events. How often should she be justified
in repeating the treatment? Should the doctor be trying something
different?**

Is this a question of 'more haste less speed?'. Look again.
Note the appearance carefully:

- Is it beefy-red, scaly, especially at the perimeter of the rash,
  with surrounding discrete sometimes pustular satellite lesions –
  all highly indicative of fungus especially monilia?

In which case focus your guns – use antifungals alone, with a
course of oral nystatin – and continue until the skin has
completely returned to a normal texture. Just a few mycelia
remaining may rapidly exacerbate when the treatment stops short.
A broader spectrum antifungal clotrimazole or miconazole might
prove more effective.

- Does the rash have a linear edge corresponding to the nappy
  margin? Is there a 'burnt' like appearance sparing the inguinal

folds? In places of prolonged contact is there ulceration? All are highly suggestive of a contact dermatitis.

In which case, increase nappy changing, bath in emollient for short periods twice a day, avoid occlusive overpants, apply protective barrier ointments (zinc, castor oil, silicone) or neutralizing benzalkonium chloride cream. Hydrocortisone 1% should help clear such a rash quickly. There can, however, be no real harm in using combinations, as fungal infection is often superadded to a basic chemical dermatitis. Babies' bottoms are wet, warm and welcoming to organisms and vulnerable to the ravages of ammonia released by urea-splitting germs and recurrences are inevitable.

Beware of severe examples. Is the mother depressed, psychotic or neglectful? Is the baby atopic, needing further exploration of the management of his/her eczema? Could this be a rare case of psoriasis?

Question 87.   Is a bath necessary?

A single-parent lady with multiple sclerosis has difficulty in managing her baby in the bath. Granny says that babies should have a bath at least 3 times a week. How often does a baby need a bath? What harm will it come to if it has none at all?

The mother should be enabled to enjoy bathing the baby.

If the mother herself has a bath sometime – aided or unaided – the baby could go in with her carried in a custom made, safe, drip-dry papoose/sling. Plastic wheelchairs can be steered or pushed under easily controlled showerheads and a baby would adapt to that too. I am sure we all need to wash away something, whether odour, secretions or cares. (We would have to ensure the baby isn't thrown out with the bathwater!)

I cannot prove a bathless baby would come to harm and I cannot justify a frequency but such a mother could always rely on me offering to bath her baby for her occasionally.

Immunization

Question 88.   Should immunization be delayed in the premature child?

A child aged 8 weeks is brought to a '6 week' child development clinic. The mother tells the doctor that the child was 8
weeks premature and that she does not want him to have his
immunizations 'until he is strong enough'. How do you modify
immunization schedules for a premature infant. . . or would you
not?

I would not.

Birthday age (see Question 43) applies here; ignore the premature weeks. There were concerns in the past about the preterm
infant's ability to mount an adequate immune response and also
concern about the IgA in breast milk interfering with oral polio
vaccine response. Neither of these in fact happen. The more pre-
term the infant, the greater the need to protect against infection,
especially pertussis and especially if the infant has any ventilator,
lung disease (bronchopulmonary dysplasia). So, convince the
mother that his lack of strength requires 'protection not rejection
from injection'.

Question 89.   When is a bad reaction truly a bad reaction?

A doctor is confronted by a lady who says that her child had a
'very bad reaction' to his first triple injection. On further
questioning it transpires that the child had a fretful night and
developed a pyrexia of 101°F. The arm was red to an area approximately 2 × 3 cm. The next day the child was better. The doctor
says that the reaction was within normal limits and advises that
the child continue with the course. Is he right? If he is, what
degree of reaction, would you say, should have influenced him to
modify the course?

This is a perfectly acceptable reaction.

His advice is correct, as all the features described are well
researched and do not constitute any elements of a severe
reaction which are:

- Local – extensive erythema and swelling over most of the antero-lateral thigh or most of the circumference of the upper arm (paper money size – not coin size).
- General – (i) Fever 39.5°C (103°F) within 48 h.
            (ii) Severe neurological events:
                - Hypotonia.
                - Unresponsiveness.
                - Prolonged, unremitting screaming.
                - Convulsions.

all within 72 hours of the injection.

            (iii) any suggestion of anaphylaxis (rare)
                - Rapidly appearing urticaria.
                - Angioneurotic oedema.
                - Hoarseness or stridor.
                - Bronchospasm.
                - Collapse.

all occurring within less than 24 hours of the injection.

Question 90. Toddlers and typhoid protection

The parents of a small toddler prone to febrile convulsions are going on holiday to a luxury hotel in the eastern Mediterranean. They say that the area is 'advised' for typhoid immunization. What advice should the doctor give? What if the child were going to a Third World country where typhoid was endemic? What general advice would you give on the holiday immunization of very small children?

If in doubt seek advice from the expert.

This child with a history of more than one convulsion has a low seizural threshold and any vaccine with a known significantly high incidence of 'reactive' fever must be carefully evaluated for advantages over disadvantages. At the time of writing the new typhoid vaccine (with little systemic effect) has become available, offering an alternative to the monovalent whole cell antigen with its high incidence of systemic reactions. However, antibody responses to the new capsular polysaccharide vaccine may be suboptimal. Oral (live) typhoid vaccine is not suitable for this age group (under 6 years).

The disease is not particularly rampant unless someone fouls the drinking water and careful hygiene, boiling drinking water, washing fruit and vegetables can be as protective as a vaccine. In a relatively low risk area I would opt not to vaccinate, but in

venturing to the Third World the balance is different. Vi polysaccharide typhoid vaccine 0.5 ml i.m. or deep s.c. can be used. If you
have to use the 'old' whole cell vaccine, prophylactic rectal
diazepam (5 mg) should be given 12 hourly (see Question 6) starting as soon as the fever begins (usually within 4 hours and lasting
24–36 h). I often seek guidance from experts at the London
School of Tropical Medicine and Hygiene's Medical Advisory
Services for Travellers Abroad (MASTA) (071 631 4408). An
excellent telephone advice about immunization needs for
travellers and their children updated with knowledge of
epidemics, unusual infections, etc. allow them to produce a
'personalized' schedule which takes the itinerary and local factors
into account, e.g. spread of cholera, Japanese B-encephalitis,
resistant malaria etc.

My general message would always be to vaccinate against
disease wherever possible, but that does not allow doctors to do
so without a thorough check of an individual's pros and cons.

Question 91.   Should live vaccine be given to chicken pox contacts?

**A child of 12 months comes to the clinic for his first MMR
immunization. His brother and sister both have chicken pox. He
has not yet had it. Is there any hazard in giving a live vaccine to
someone who is very likely incubating another virus infection?
What if he were to have polio vaccination in these circumstances?**

Delay for a short while.

A history of contact with an infectious disease is not a
contraindication to the use of MMR, or polio vaccine. In truth
superimposed viral infections must be a frequent occurrence,
spontaneously or iatrogenically, and unrecognized in most circumstances. Thus the risks are very low.

The varicella virus is capable of causing marked immunosup-
pressive effects which probably account for the so-called
'secondary' bacterial infections frequent after chicken pox, e.g.
otitis media, late pneumonia and infected skin lesions. I cannot
see the point of indecent haste in the situation described and I
would wait until the child finished his chicken pox (or waiting no
more than 4 weeks if he refused to incubate) before immunization with MMR (or polio). The only circumstance that might
change my mind would be if the immediate community were in
the throes of a measles or mumps epidemic – then, I would
immunize early.

Question 92. Is there a 'best site' for infant injections?

Is there any chosen injection site that for reasons of reduction of local reaction, safety and effectiveness, is preferred to any other?

Buttock is best.

The official guide to good immunization (DOH) counsels that immunizing injections (other than those intended intradermal, e.g. BCG) are given as i.m. or deep subcutaneous injections. The favoured sites are the antero-lateral aspect of the thigh and the upper arm (deltoid region).

Factors to be considered are given in Table 9.

Until 5 years ago, I was a devotee of the thigh. Local reactions and subcutaneous fat damage are not infrequently seen on thighs and upper arms. The passionate exhortations of a GP who had diligently audited the reactions he had seen and who adamantly believed that 'bum was best' finally convinced me to use the buttock. It is vital to site the injection correctly and deeply. The baby or child, prone on the couch, held by the ipsilateral knee is relaxed at the time of the injection. (Readers would wish to be assured that I regularly immunize children, but not in large numbers).

Table 9. Best site for infant injections

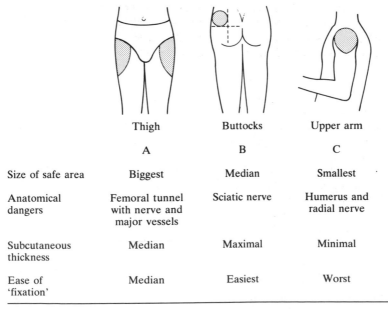

	Thigh	Buttocks	Upper arm
	A	B	C
Size of safe area	Biggest	Median	Smallest
Anatomical dangers	Femoral tunnel with nerve and major vessels	Sciatic nerve	Humerus and radial nerve
Subcutaneous thickness	Median	Maximal	Minimal
Ease of 'fixation'	Median	Easiest	Worst

N.B. Hepatitis B vaccine must *not* be given into buttock fat.

Question 93. Whooping cough vaccine and family convulsions

A woman comes to the 8-week immunization clinic with her baby. She says that she does not want her child to have Pertussis vaccine because both her sisters have children who had convulsions following such immunization. The doctor says that this is no contraindication and says that not to have it would be neglectful. Is he treading on thin ice if anything goes wrong?

The doctor is right but extra support may be required.

First cousins are not first degree relatives and the genetic link to febrile or non-febrile fits does not therefore exist here. Only the parents or the baby's own siblings would be relevant. DPT vaccine may cause fever in as many as 50% of infants (with some 6% reaching >39°C) within 48 hours of the injection. With febrile convulsions occurring in 2–3% of children under the age of 5 years – although very few of these occur under 6 months of age – there is bound to be a fit 'by chance' within 48 hours of some injections. The risk of damage from a convulsion directly connected to the injection or by random coincidence is extremely small.

The doctor has to communicate with confidence and conviction but must sense the degree of proper anxiety. The relationship of the time of the convulsion to the time of the injection in the cousins is vital to know and think about. Prophylactic paracetamol 10–15 mg/kg per dose (at this age) can be given at the time of the injection and 4–6 hourly for up to 72 hours. This has been shown to work in reducing the risk of high fever after immunization. This is an acceptable alternative to giving 60 mg (if aged 2–3 months) of paracetamol liquid **ONLY** if a post-immunization pyrexia appears, to be repeated once later (4–6 hours) if indicated.

Finally, I always offer to perform any 'doubter's' jabs in the hospital with a stay for 24 hours (or longer if symptoms appear). This is often only necessary for the first jab and the parents' confidence usually improves with proper support. High immunization rates depend on extra support for those with anxiety in order to win over doubters and stop rumours undermining our best endeavours.

Question 94. Is *Haemophilus influenzae* vaccination hazardous?

Are there any hazards involved in *Haemophilus influenzae* immunization? What are the conditions it is likely to prevent?

It is safe and prevents a variety of extremely nasty infections.

It has been estimated that annually, in the UK there are about 1300 cases of *H. influenzae* type b disease, 900 cases of meningitis caused by this organism and 65 deaths that might be largely preventable in the under 5s by immunization. Extrapolating figures from the Oxford study, epiglottitis (as lethal as meningitis) – 150 cases, osteomyelitis – 80 cases, pneumonia, cellulitis and bacteraemia all due to this micro organism are preventable each year.

Three injections are given at 2, 3 and 4 months of age, at the same time, but in a separate site to the DPT vaccine. Oral polio vaccine goes along too. The Finns are trying a combined quadrivalent vaccine (I don't know if they are just kinder, wiser or stingier!) Local reactions (2%) seem to be much fewer than from the DPT vaccine (in which some 20% have a reaction greater than 2 cm). General reactions such as fever >38°C (5%), irritability lasting longer than 4 hours (23%), or inconsolable crying for >1 hour occurred at the same sort of frequency as with DPT vaccine. Febrile convulsions are said to have no higher incidence than with DPT alone.

Miscellaneous

Question 95. Is cot death a recurrent condition?

The parents of a new-born baby approach their doctor asking for an apnoea alarm as their first child died in a 'cot death' situation at 6 months. They are extremely anxious. How should they be counselled? Are they more likely, less likely or as likely, compared to other parents, to be faced with another such tragedy?

There is just under twice the chance that a family who have suffered a cot death will have a recurrence of the tragedy compared to a family who have not. But the overall incidence, and thus the risk, is falling rapidly.

One hopes that at the time of the first tragedy the parents and siblings were handled with great sensitivity, were allowed to grieve, were supported by all the available agencies and all relevant information was made available – including the post-mortem result which may, or may not, have explained the cause of death. An early further pregnancy, attempting to avoid mourning or unresolved grief, should have been counselled against. Most families take 6–12 months to reconstruct themselves. Promoting positive feelings for the new baby needs a lot of work antenatally, clarifying new anxieties and inevitably discussing the latest explanations for sudden infant death, particularly the new guide lines. This is the time to discuss the use of an apnoea alarm and to demonstrate its use.

Continuation of care involves checking the baby immediately at birth and offering close, reliable access to familiar (and trusted) medical advice which GP, health visitor and consultant paediatricians should share. Emotional support might be found from a Sudden Infant Death Syndrome (SIDS) foundation member if the parents have sought such a liaison.

The vexed issue of apnoea alarm support involves an open and honest résumé of all pros and cons, the final choice being left to the parents. Should they choose to proceed they need immediate training on the technicalities of the device, as well as how to resuscitate in the face of an arrest.

Anxieties, whatever the degree of support, rise to a crescendo at the time the new infant reaches the age at which the previous child died. Thereafter confidence grows as time distances them from this fearsome watershed. Reported at an incidence of 1 in 450 live births (LB) in England and Wales in 1985–87, with the chance of 'recurrence' in the same family about double, i.e. 1 in 250 LB, we can happily report that as we write now there has been considerable reduction in deaths from SIDS over the last 2–3 years.

We cannot be certain of the reasons why but perhaps the following may be of help:

* The adoption of lateral or supine sleep positions and NOT PRONE LYING.
* The avoidance of overheating or overwrapping.
* The early recognition of disease by parents, e.g. baby-check system and health care workers.
* The impact of educational propaganda – to breast feed, reduce passive smoking, etc.
* The screening for metabolic disease where an appropriate history, e.g. fatty acidopathy, is combining to make effective inroads into reducing the commonest cause of infant deaths from the age of 1 week to 1 year.

Question 96.   Are chloramphenicol eye drops dangerous?

A highly intelligent mother brings her small infant son to the doctor with conjunctivitis. As the doctor is writing out a prescription for chloramphenicol eye drops the mother comments that her father recently suffered an asthma attack following administration, and absorption, of beta blocker eye drops for his glaucoma. 'There's nothing in these drops that could possibly harm my baby is there?' she asks. How should the doctor reply? Are chloramphenicol eye drops and eye ointment safe?

These products are safe.

A line has to be drawn somewhere. The risk, theoretical, is infinitely small. The total chloramphenicol content of the eye ointment (4 g of 1%) and the eye drops (10 ml of ½%) is 40 mg and 50 mg of chloramphenicol, respectively. Only a tiny proportion of this small amount, even if all were used, would find its way down the nasolacrimal duct. My reply to the mother, assuming that the conjunctivitis required treatment with chloramphenicol (and was not chlamydial nor, simply, the sticky eye of a blocked nasolacrimal duct requiring only gentle cleaning with sterile water) would be to say it was the best, safest way I had to protect such an important part of the baby's body.

Question 97. Heart murmur. Breaking the news

At a 6-week medical examination a baby seems perfectly well. The doctor examining the child finds a soft, systolic bruit at the left sternal edge. The mother is under treatment for severe post-natal depression. How should the doctor proceed?

With honesty and as much reassurance as possible.

Statistically, the commonest cause of a murmur at this stage of development is a ventricular septal defect (VSD), and the signs described would be compatible. If a VSD, the louder the murmur, the smaller the defect. A confident experienced (in paediatric cardiac matters) GP may feel he can diagnose the straightforward VSDs and wish to put off any discussion or referral until the mother improves, or a better opportunity arises. I think such an approach would be precarious. A little forethought, so often done by health visitors, should ensure the attendance of father or close supporter of the mother, when routine checks on a baby of a severely depressed woman are to occur.

If there are important signs and symptoms, the infant's needs are just as important as those of the mother. If the mother were alone I would keep her in the surgery while contacting her partner, closely involved member of the family/friend, or her health care worker, e.g. community psychiatric nurse. I would share the idea that a paediatric or paediatric cardiologist's opinion is needed, emphasizing that:

- The chances of a serious problem are minimal.
- Early diagnosis of even complicated cardiac anomalies now carries a high probability of total remedy.

I favour telling the truth within the limit of ability, ensuring the best outcome for the infant's condition and maximum support for the mother. I am sure, in these circumstances, in order to minimize anxiety for the mother, the local paediatrician would see the child within a very short time.

Question 98. Expectations and Down's syndrome

In a large practice there are several patients with Down's syndrome. They vary from the extremely dependent and handicapped to one who reads and writes, is most responsible and holds down an unskilled job. Is there any indication early on that might

suggest which children will do better than others? Is high expectation a spur to maximizing performance or is it a major source of acute disappointment and frustration?

Everything that can hold back a normal child will hold back a Down's child more.

Down's syndrome children are recognized by similar physical features and deportment. When you are involved with caring for them as a health worker over a period of time it is equally apparent that they have infinite differences. The damage wreaked by the extra genetic material on chromosome 21 must obviously be modified by the interplay of the remaining genes and other nurturing events:

- *The amount of extra 21 genetic material.* Regular Down's (94%) brings three sets of that chromosome's genes, but translocations (3.5%) and mosaicism (2.5%) give a very different balance and often a very different order of abnormalities or handicap. Associated anomalies are rife, with almost 50% having cardiac defects and up to 10% significant bowel anomalies. It would not be surprising to expect the brain structure, anatomical or functional, to show such variation.
- *The modifications of 'normal' genes.* Skin pigment, hair colour, height and muscular strength can all be seen as different and easily matched to parental characteristics. There must be similar influences on intelligence too.
- *The impact of severe, associated anomalies.* Severe cardiac disease, frequent chest infection, hypothyroidism, etc. may lead to long periods of hospitalization or curtailed activity and learning opportunity. These would affect any child's progress, but the handicapped child is the greater loser. As a simple concept, losing 2–3 points off your potential when it is 100 is half as bad as losing 2–3 points off a potential of 50. Deafness (usually middle ear disease but occasionally sensori-neural), poor vision (33% have squints, 15% nystagmus, 1% cataracts), many refractive errors – are all so frequent that they pile on the agony of handicapping factors to the Down's learning potential.
- *The psychodynamic effects on the family.* The grief responses in a family faced with the devastation of having a severely handicapped child show wide variation. The courage and strengths of individuals, the power of support or failure of family relationships, the positive or negative interaction with healthcare professionals are just some of the features that may play a vital part in the early and subsequent development of these stricken children.

Experience shows the more rapidly responses are constructively worked through and the depression effectively lifted, the less effect on the child's progress. There may be critical windows for learning and development and thus permanent damage may ensue during these most stressful times. The greater our enlightenment about all these dynamics the more our Down's children may be helped to achieve.

• *Society's response.* Radical changes in attitudes, availability of professional expertise, facilities to share the burden of handicap, acceptance of the child whatever the appearance and disability into a normal integrated lifestyle and positive discrimination regarding resources, will all move mountains in alleviating the negative aspects of development that might otherwise predominate. There has been a lot of progress but current reforms in social services, health and education have yet to be tested as to whether the child with special needs is to be an overall winner or loser.

There can be no doubt that the historical assessments of Down's children's intellectual potential were wrong and reflected the total impact of many adverse factors discussed, a lot of which are amenable to remedy. There is clearly irreparable limitations to their IQ (except a few rare mosaics or milder translocations). No regular Down's child is likely to achieve a performance score much in excess of 70, but used to its fullest, with good physical social and behavioural skills, 70 can be a very 'independent state of being'. Self-care, social integration, and work potential albeit of a sheltered nature should thus be possible. If all stages of this latency are happy, fulfilled and encouraged – by no means easy – the child's potential will be reached. Major difficulties still exist in written and language skills. There is a high incidence of hypothyroidism over time and an Alzheimer-like dementia may frequently curtail achievement and life expectancy, quite apart from severe anomalies of the heart.

Not all Down's children have such good potential and are 'programmed' for severe learning difficulties rather than moderate or mild. The development of Down's children follows normal sequences, but at a slower pace and the final threshold of achievement is going to be only two-thirds normal. Skilful developmental observation and recording in the early months (up to a year) should give a straightforward velocity chart of achievement and point to the worst versus the best achievers. Speed of motor development, as in normal children, is not a good predictor of IQ. Alertness, attention span and manipulative skills all yield better signals of potential. Language can be disproportionately bad and adversely affect achievement. Language is best gauged throughout the second year.

Question 99. Allergic to penicillin?

A boy of 6 years, with tonsillitis, is brought to the doctor by his mother. The family is new to the area. The GP is about to prescribe penicillin when the mother says 'He's allergic to penicillin, Doctor, The last time it was given to him, he came out in a rash'. How likely is it that the child is truly allergic to penicillin? Should the doctor ignore what happened previously and prescribe penicillin?

Though the child is unlikely to be allergic to penicillin it should not be prescribed in these circumstances.

Penicillin is very commonly given for upper respiratory infections in children, although the majority of such episodes – perhaps 90% – are viral. By their nature these infections frequently produce exanthemata. Penicillin ingestion, therefore, very often coincides with a rash in circumstances where the two factors are not related. Several good studies on 'alleged' penicillin allergy have shown a low incidence of proven reaction using a combination of scrupulous history taking, skin tests, in vitro RAST tests and challenges.

It is possible for penicillin to cause severe reactions such as anaphylactic shock, the Stevens–Johnson syndrome, or even a vasculitic reaction with urticaria, raised purpura and haemorrhagic blisters. These reactions are all rare.

The most common type of penicillin reaction is a widespread symmetrical, mostly truncal morbilliform reaction. It is more often of sudden onset, associated with itching and with little or mild fever initially. The child will often feel unwell in a non-specific way. Arthralgia and even florid arthropathy especially in large joints may appear if the drug continues. The interval between drug and initial onset of rash is often 7–10 days unless the child has been exposed to and reacted to the drug previously. Most drug rashes will persist or worsen as long as the drug is taken. The rash usually disperses rapidly when the agent is withdrawn. Urticarial rashes raise the likelihood of drug origin, but these, too, may be viral or non-drug in origin. Cross-reactivity between penicillins and cephalosporins is not well understood and should not be assumed (but when systemic antibiotics may be vital for a life-threatening infection, considerable caution will need to be applied).

When this child has recovered from his tonsillitis I would think it worth finding out whether or not he was truly allergic to penicillin. I would rather see a child in out-patients than have him landed with an assumed diagnosis that might have some serious significance with a future, severe bacterial infection. I might

RAST test against penicillin but the history would be the most important and if there was any doubt I would be prepared to give a small amount of oral penicillin, e.g. Pen.V 125 mg, under close supervision, preferably in hospital. Provided no immediate reaction occurred, after 48 hours, I would give a dose of 250 mg orally. No reaction, early or late, after 2 weeks, would lead me to mark the boy down as not allergic to penicillin.

Nevertheless, in the particular circumstances, posed in this question, to carry on and prescribe penicillin, willy-nilly, when you have been told the child is allergic courts disaster. Either reassure the mother that 80% of tonsillitis is viral or, if she insists an antibiotic is needed, use erythromycin. You might even persuade her to wait while a throat swab gave 'scientific' choices.

Question 100.   Child abuse? The need for sensitivity

The 8-year-old daughter of a 'pillar of society' is brought by both her parents to see the GP. She has a history of vague abdominal pain and is said by her mother to 'cry easily'. The GP has been alerted by a very sensitive school nurse that there might be a possibility of sexual abuse by the father. Should the doctor ask to see the child without her parents being present? If he does, should he have a chaperone? What are the factors in a child's demeanour that lead you to suspect sexual abuse?

The parents should be present during the examination. There can be many clues in the child's demeanour.

The investigation of suspected child sexual abuse (CSA) requires the doctor to be a skilful detective, but with a motive for help and understanding, rather than conviction and punishment. There is an area child protection committee with a GP member which publishes and distributes guidelines for all agencies when confronted by this sort of problem. The name, location telephone number and role of all appropriate local expertise is available in this booklet. Any person suspicious of child abuse should contact the child protection team (CPT) who offer a 24-hour service and will respond immediately. There is usually an *initial strategy meeting* (often held at a GPs practice) and in this case an experienced social worker and a trained police officer would meet the school nurse involved, probably the school headmistress or delegated teacher, yourself and perhaps the family's health visitor. Your collective knowledge of the family and the evidence would almost certainly bring an important bearing on the way forward.

If the substance of the concern seems substantial it might prove wiser to hand over to the CPT with immediate involvement of a skilled child protection doctor. In our district a number of GPs are trained for this role.

But suppose you did not forearm yourself in this way. As it is more and more likely CSA concerns may arise out of many unexpected situations, all GPs must have a clinical approach to children and their families that prepares them for coping with the unpredictable. Remember:

* Abusing parents have little or no insight into their behaviour.
* Powerful forces of denial are at work, in both the perpetrator and the rest of the family (most CSA occurs within the family). There are few opportunities for confessions – probabilities rather than certainties are the usual conclusions.
* The complexity of psychopathological mechanisms within the family never allows quick and easy conclusions to be drawn.

I would suggest a routine clinical approach be pursued with careful history, examination and observation. There should be no need to arouse suspicions in the parents. Unfortunately, the examination of children has now become 'tainted' because of adverse publicity surrounding the Cleveland cases. I have always examined genitalia and I do not intend to be hounded out of a sound and proper clinical practice. I constantly find important pathology, totally unrelated to concerns about CSA, which establishes a correct diagnosis and directs specific therapy, e.g. fused labia causing recurrent urinary tract infection or vulvovaginitis; threadworms; fissure in ano; congenital ano/urethral anomalies; inguinal hernias, etc. It is imperative that all doctors learn how to achieve a child's (and parents) approval for examination of any part of his/her anatomy. Here are some practical hints:

* I always recognize the child's right to consent, explaining what I want to examine and why. I use words appropriate to the child's level of understanding and his/her social/cultural background. I often opt to do this via the parent, who can explain in their own intimate language (literal/figurative use of the word language). How the parent does this is often revealing. It is vital to establish the child's names and understanding when referring to the genitalia and anus.
* I would always ask a reticent child whether they would prefer a lady doctor (as a male doctor myself) to examine them – recognizing the possibilities of cultural taboos as well as personal preference, quite apart from the knowledge that perpetrators of CSA are mostly male.
* I always emphasize to children that they must never let themselves be examined by a stranger. I explain that only if their parent or parents are present would they know who was

a real doctor, and only real doctors can help mum/dad find out what the pain or illness is due to. I usually tell young children that doctors are 'nosey-parkers' who try to find all the clues they can to work out the puzzle. I would *never* examine a child without a parent present. These are all rules to avoid confusing the child's knowledge of acceptable behaviour and previous 'child protection' training.

- Only the parents, or a nurse helping a parent, should undress a child if he/she cannot manage. I only examine the genitalia in a logical sequence, never first, never the only part examined – usually after examining the abdomen and back. I explain to the child (and parents) why I need to see their private parts and I inform them that I will not touch anything without their consent. It is usually better for them to show the parts themselves, or I ask the parent to do all the manipulating and holding. It becomes quick and easy once you have perfected the communication techniques.
- Never ask leading questions, but non-directed ones such as 'did something happen to hurt you here' or 'do you remember anything that might have made this bit (e.g. 'front bum') sore'. Record your exact question and the answers given. How the child handles this whole examination and responds to the open questions needs to be carefully observed and recorded.

While you are working through this process you will be mindful of the manifestations of sexual abuse. These can be considered as:

- The physical manifestations (not detailed here):
  - Anogenital injuries and diseases.
  - Lesions elsewhere, mouth, breasts, thighs and buttocks, lower abdomen.
  - (Teenage pregnancy in an older child).

- The behavioural manifestations:
  - Sexual activity acted out in words, play or written work may reveal the events and may preoccupy the abused child.
  - Precocious sexual acts may occur in a child of this age, with seductive and 'street-wise' behaviour.
  - Regressive behaviour especially soiling and wetting appearing for the first time or relapsing.
  - Altered feeding patterns – bulimia or anorexia.
  - Withdrawn behaviour and social isolation.
  - Falling school performance.
  - Truancy, hysteria, drug abuse (alcohol, glue-sniffing etc.).
  - Self mutilation.
  - Suicidal attempts.

I would not attempt to see the child on her own, but I might see the parents without the child. Unless strong evidence has emerged, my questions to parents would be open and non-confrontational, and I would always try to be informative to parents. You may need to leave a path open for a further opinion – a situation that is a straightforward process for most GPs. The child's needs must be carefully thought about, and always share doubts with the specialists you work with (hopefully your local friendly paediatrician). Remember the 'processes of child abuse' are such that wrong moves at the beginning may make it harder for the child to 'disclose' or put the perpetrators more on their guard.

116

Index

Index number refers to question number